Orthodox and Alternative Medicine

Orthodox and Alternative Medicine

Politics, Professionalization and Health Care

MIKE SAKS

SAGE Publications
London • Thousand Oaks • New Delhi

SAGE Publications Ltd
6 Bonhill Street
London EC2A 4PU

SAGE Publications Inc
2455 Teller Road
Thousand Oaks, California 91320

SAGE Publications India Pvt Ltd
32, M-Block Market
Greater Kailash – 1
New Delhi 110 048

British Library Cataloguing-in-Publication Data
A catalogue record for this book is available from the British Library.

ISBN 1–4129–0153–7

Library of Congress Cataloging-in-Publication Data

Saks, Mike.
    Orthodox and alternative medicine: politics, professionalization, and health care/Mike Saks.
        p. cm.
    Includes bibliographical references and index.
    ISBN 0–8264–5817–3 – ISBN 0–8264–5818–1 (pb.)
    1. Medicine–Great Britain–History. 2. Alternative medicine–Great Britain–History.
    I. Title

R487 .S354 2002
362.1'0941–dc21   2002071607

Typeset by BookEns Ltd, Royston, Herts
Printed and bound in Great Britain by Athenaeum Press Ltd., Gateshead

Contents

Acknowledgements

Acknowledgements go to the many colleagues, too numerous to name, who have discussed with me the various areas covered by this book over many years, in national and international conferences, symposia and other forums. Most of all, though, thanks go to my family – my wife Maj-Lis and my children Jonathan and Laura – who through their tolerance of my twilight activities as an author and researcher have made this book possible.

Introduction

The Introduction will set the scene for the volume by placing the study of the development of orthodox and alternative medicine in its wider context and outlining the mainstream concepts on which it is based. The main focus of the book is on the social scientific analysis of the fascinating historical and contemporary relationship between orthodox medicine and alternative medicine in Britain and the United States. The differences in the underlying socio-political framework of British and American society are fully acknowledged in this process – including the more decentralized political system of the United States as compared with that of Britain (Blondel 1995). As will be seen in this book, such distinctions have influenced the form that the interface between orthodox and unorthodox medicine has taken in these countries. The differences are particularly apparent in relation to the notion of professionalization, which – having once been exclusively linked to orthodox health care – is now increasingly also becoming associated with practitioners of the medical alternatives, from acupuncturists to osteopaths.

The case of professionalization also provides a salutary reminder that there are similarities as well as differences between Britain and the United States. Aside from the fact that both countries are normally identified as capitalist, it is often argued that the development of professional groups is distinctive to these societies in the more advanced industrial world. In this respect, the Anglo-American context is differentiated from much of continental Europe, where there is a less marked tradition of professional independence in the occupational sector (Collins 1990). This is certainly true of state centralist societies like France and countries in the former Soviet empire where groups such as doctors and nurses were subordinated to the perceived interests of the party and the socialist state. However, given that there are gradations in the extent of professional autonomy in Europe and significant distinctions in the nature of professions even within Britain and the United States, there is a strong case for viewing the professional standing of occupations as lying on a spectrum. On this continuum, the location of any specific group is based on its level of independence at the point in time at which it is being considered (Macdonald 1995).

The notion of there being a continuum – the form of which may change over time – rather than a stark polarity of types is also helpful in understanding the concepts of orthodox and alternative medicine, which are pivotal to this volume. Orthodox medicine is seen here as encompassing those forms of health care in the division of labour that are to a significant extent formally underwritten by the state. At present, such orthodoxy in the contemporary Anglo-American context is based on biomedicine, a framework for practice largely centred on the use of drugs and surgery (Saks 1992a). In modern times, biomedical orthodoxy has been responsible for many developments, from penicillin to plastic surgery (Duffin 1999). It is also changing very rapidly – with current advances ranging from the use of genetic engineering and magnetic resonance imaging to organ transplantation and micro-surgery (Le Fanu 1999). There is not, however, an inextricable link between the biomedical paradigm and medical orthodoxy. Even though they have been synonymous for the past century or more in Britain and the United States, such associations can change as time progresses.

By the same token, neither is alternative medicine as defined in this book inevitably based on the wide range of therapies that are at present typically included in this field. In this regard, alternative medicine is not even seen as constituting a single approach with a common philosophy, for there are many variations between the dozens of such therapies available today in Britain and the United States. At one end of the spectrum, they encompass acupuncture and aromatherapy, based on the therapeutic use of needles and essential plant oils respectively. At the other, there are therapies such as homoeopathy, centred on giving extreme dilutions of remedies and the principle that 'like cures like', and different types of manipulation of the spine and other joints embodied in chiropractic and osteopathy (see, for example, Stanway 1994; Bruce and McIlwain 1998). The diversity of this field in the Anglo-American context is underlined by the many categories into which such therapies have been divided by authors on this subject. These span from creative, sensory, mind–body and manual therapies (Fulder 1996) to clinical, psychological/ behavioural and social/community forms of therapy (Kelner and Wellman 2000).

The very breadth of the provision indicates the limitations of analyses that try to define the field in terms of its substantive characteristics. The concept of 'traditional medicine', for example, does not cover recently developed areas such as biofeedback, in which subjects employ technical instrumentation to self-monitor their mental states. The term 'complementary medicine', moreover, may omit therapies such as homoeopathy that are based on philosophical principles fundamentally counterposed to those of biomedical orthodoxy. The notion of 'holistic medicine', on the other hand, is by no means the exclusive domain of alternative practitioners and does not necessarily apply to groups such as osteopaths who use their methods mechanistically simply to treat bad backs (Saks 1992a). Similar caveats apply to attempts to pin down orthodox medicine too precisely, given the great variations, and sometimes contradictions, in approach that occur between biomedical practices – not least in cross-cultural settings in advanced industrial societies (Payer 1990).

Just as 'medical orthodoxy' is defined here on the basis of its political legitimacy, therefore, 'alternative medicine' is conceived in terms of its political marginality. This is accentuated by, among other things, the limited support the latter has generally received from official sources of research funding, its typical exclusion from the mainstream medical curriculum, its less than positive representation in the major medical journals, and the formal restrictions imposed on its practice (Saks 1995b). Thus the definitions of orthodox and alternative medicine that underpin this volume are relative. In this sense, the mainstream practices of one era in any particular country may become the unorthodoxy of another, and vice versa, a fact that throws into focus the politics of defining orthodox and alternative medicine. Whatever the current relative standing of orthodox biomedicine and the medical alternatives in British and American society, it is not assumed here that the associated patterns of dominance and exclusion are necessarily objectively derived from the 'scientific' or 'non-scientific' status of the knowledge involved (Saks 1998a). Indeed, the notion that Western science is distinctively based on 'objective' truth has been effectively debunked by the work of philosophers such as Popper (1963) and Kuhn (1970). They have variously underlined the provisional nature of all knowledge and pointed to the framework of assumptions within which even 'normal' science is conducted.

It can therefore no longer be reasonably claimed that there are universally accepted rules of the scientific game that make orthodox Western science a neutral and epistemologically privileged activity compared to alternative ways of understanding the world – as was once confidently pronounced by social theorists (see, for instance, Merton 1968). There are, however, other means of analysing both sides of the health-care coin in a more relativistic manner. In this respect, orthodox and unorthodox medicine are studied here in terms of the politics of work, within a neo-Weberian frame of reference. This perspective places a particular emphasis on examining the interplay of competing occupational group interests within the wider socio-economic order. In this framework, successful occupations are seen as gaining increased income, status and power in the marketplace by socially excluding their competitors, who conversely lose out in the struggle for such rewards (Saks 1995b). This approach, focused on relationships of domination and subordination, centrally underlies the notion of professionalization, which is viewed as pivotal to the historical and contemporary analysis of health care in Britain and the United States.

On this basis, the book questions the traditional social scientific view of trait and functionalist writers on professions as necessarily centred on unique bodies of specialized expertise of great value to society, employed in the interests of clients and/or the wider public (see Millerson 1964). In contrast, professionalization is defined in more in-vogue neo-Weberian terms as being based on the establishment of patterns of legally underwritten exclusionary social closure, gained by some occupations in the politics of work. Although such closure is also typically seen as being founded on a lengthy period of education and subscription to ethical codes, it is crucially held to involve the formation of professional monopolies over socio-economic opportunities that directly or indirectly exclude occupational rivals operating in the market. This exclusion is viewed as occurring in a political process in which professional claims about such matters as the esoteric knowledge they employ and their distinctive public service orientation must be critically examined, and cannot simply be taken at face value (see Saks 1998b).

From this viewpoint, it is argued that such claims can be seen as strategically employed ideologies that maintain or further the interests of the group(s) concerned – resulting in more fully fledged professions gaining the support of the state. There are many debates about the meaning of the notion of 'interests'. As it is so central to the arguments pursued in this book, it is worth reflecting – as discussed by Saks (1995b) – that the definitions of this concept in the literature are theoretically wide-ranging. Some are rooted in the positivist approach, which sees interests as subjective policy preferences that are more or less overtly expressed by the groups concerned. Others are centred on the realist perspective, which holds that interests are not directly observable as they are subject to the distorting influence of dominant ideologies. In this context, however, the concept of interests is defined in terms of the conventionalist approach as being furthered when there is an objective improvement in the collective position of a group based on the balance of costs and benefits, in terms of income, status and power. This has the advantage of being both tangible and operational in considering the interplay between politics, professionalization and health care in Britain and the United States.

In terms of professionalization, the occupational group that has obtained one of the most privileged, autonomous positions in the marketplace in the contemporary Anglo-American context is that of medicine, the current standing of which is paralleled only by that of law (Macdonald 1995).

Exclusionary forms of social closure, though, are by no means restricted to these classic professions – with licensure extending to groups as diverse as architects and accountants in Britain and the United States (Macdonald 1985; Freidson 1986). In the health field, the professionalization of medicine in both these countries has been associated with the establishment of a range of subordinated allied professions, sometimes referred to as semi-professions, including occupations such as nursing, midwifery and pharmacy (Saks 1998b; Freidson 1994). Now a number of groups previously regarded as unorthodox, such as osteopaths and chiropractors, have also variously professionalized (Saks 1999b; Gevitz 1988a). This underlines the importance of the state underwriting claims to be a profession in the interface between orthodox and alternative medicine.

Having provided a broad conceptual framework for the study, the book develops in the following way. Focusing on Britain and the United States, Chapter 1 will describe earlier traditions of health care, highlighting the diversity of approaches on offer in the immediate pre-industrial era. It will also outline the emergence of the separate categories of orthodox and alternative medicine from a relatively undifferentiated past, in the wake of the growing move to professionalize medicine on both sides of the Atlantic. The professionalization of orthodox medical practitioners and, subsequently, allied health workers in this context will be discussed further in Chapter 2 – as well as the development up to the mid-twentieth century of orthodox biomedicine, with its growing association with science and a rapidly expanding technological base. Chapter 3 will go on to examine the marginalization of unorthodox therapies resulting from the dominance of mainstream medicine, including the implications of the increasing division between both orthodox and alternative medicine for the therapies concerned.

The limits that the generally negative medical response imposed on alternative medicine up to the mid-twentieth century have been tempered, however, by the recent resurgence of interest in unorthodox forms of health care. This was particularly fuelled in the 1960s and 1970s by the growth of a strong counter-culture in the West. After considering the key developments in orthodox and unorthodox medicine immediately following the mid-twentieth century, Chapter 4 will chart the ensuing critique of orthodox forms of health care and spiralling consumer interest in the medical alternatives. In addition, it considers the shifting response of orthodox medicine to such therapies. Chapter 5 meanwhile will explore changes in mainstream health policy from the mid-1970s onwards, including the impact of the changes on the professional standing of medicine, which has been brought into question by some commentators. This chapter also examines the increasing trend for practitioners of unorthodox therapies to professionalize in Britain and the

United States. The ramifications of this development are considered, at a time when orthodoxy itself has not stood still. Finally, the Conclusion will draw together the main threads of the argument, reflecting on the possible future relationship between orthodox and alternative medicine in the Anglo-American context – including the prospects for more integrated health care as the twenty-first century unfolds.

Societal continuities as well as discontinuities will be apparent from this discussion, particularly in relation to Britain and the United States, the countries around which the book primarily revolves. These continuities and discontinuities reflect the similarities and differences in the social context in which health care is situated in these two countries. The main argument in this volume, however, is that interest-based politics, rather than scientific logic *per se*, is central to the understanding of health care in general and the relationship between orthodox and alternative medicine in particular. This theme has underpinned the work of the present author in a number of publications elsewhere (see, for instance, Saks 1987, 1991a, 1995b). As this volume indicates, it certainly seems to apply to the past and the present, as highlighted by the turf wars surrounding professionalization. Interest-based politics also appears likely to continue to be a major force in shaping health care in all its various forms in the future.

The book builds on extensive research conducted by the author in this field over a twenty-five-year period. This volume has been written to appeal to a higher-level undergraduate and postgraduate market, as well as to academic colleagues in the social sciences interested in the development of, and interface between, orthodox and alternative medicine. In this sense, it should be of particular interest to those working in such areas as sociology, social history, social policy and politics. The intriguing material that it covers is also relevant to both practising health workers and students at an advanced stage of their training and education in the professionalized – and professionalizing – segments of the health sector, including those involved in the management of health services. It is hoped too that the book will prove helpful to current consumers of health care, as well as the general reader. They may appreciate the opportunity to place their experiences in the health field in the broader socio-political context set out in the pages that follow.

A major attraction to all these potential readers is that the book for the first time provides a balanced account of the development of health care in the Anglo-American context, an account that considers both orthodox and unorthodox medicine on a level playing field. In this sense, it avoids the one-sided narratives that have so characterized the literature on health care, which generally focus on either orthodox or alternative medicine, in some cases as if the two were entirely separate spheres. In examining both sides of the healthcare coin from an interest-based neo-Weberian perspective with a particular emphasis on the theme of professionalization, this volume provides a holistic overview of the past, present and future of health care. By considering medical orthodoxy and unorthodoxy, it is able to discuss the synergies between the two, rather than simply viewing them in abstraction. In this respect, the book aims to demonstrate the applicability to health care in Britain and the United States of the well-worn dictum that 'the whole is much greater than the sum of its parts'.

CHAPTER I

Health care in the pre-industrial era

This chapter describes the forms of health care that existed in the immediate pre-industrial era in both Britain and the United States. The time line of the start of the sixteenth century, chosen to mark the beginning of the study, is necessarily somewhat arbitrary. As Cule (1997) notes, the history of health care goes back to the start of humankind – initially usually being undertaken in the most basic fashion, with a range of traditional healers in different parts of the world, from the African witch doctor to the Siberian shaman. These complemented the largely self-administered plant treatments, religiously based therapies and other folk remedies that were variously on offer. Such patterns of health care had many different cross-cultural manifestations, including a number of key milestones in the development of modern Western medicine, on which this book is centred. Examples of these were those laid over two thousand years ago in Greece by Hippocrates, who believed that the human body should be seen as a whole and could be influenced by the wider environment – and subsequently by Galen, the famed Roman doctor who wrote on anatomy, physiology and practical medicine. Similarly strong strands in relation to the foundations of modern Western medicine were also drawn from wider geographical areas – including a thousand or so years ago from such thinkers in Arab medicine as Avicenna, who were important in teaching the practice of prescribing (Duffin 1999).

These influences, together with the power of the Church, as Duin and Sutcliffe (1992) observe, continued to affect health care throughout the Middle Ages in Western Europe. Although suffering was seen more as part of the human condition, and the classical texts were only selectively drawn upon, such practices as cupping and bloodletting to restore balance and fortify the body were perpetuated up to the Renaissance. At this time, humanist thought is held to have begun to supplant some of the earlier religious dogma in health care. Rudimentary surgery was carried out to a greater extent for a number of conditions. This humanist perspective coexisted alongside belief systems such as astrology that not only had popular currency, but also permeated the thinking of some of the emerging groups of physicians and surgeons. As a result, in medieval times in the West, there were several competing schools of thought based on differing perceived symptomatic cures – including those involving herbal remedies and dietetics, among others. Their delivery by practitioners was increasingly based on teaching in the emerging universities as well as on the far more common apprenticeship model, with the precise treatment administered largely reflecting the wishes of particular clients in a predominantly fee-for-service system (Cule 1997).

As we shall see, North America was also affected by the Western European experience, starting with the initial impact of explorers, missionaries and soldiers from countries such as Spain, France and England. They came into contact with the culture of the various North American Indian tribes from the late fifteenth century onwards. At this time, the sparsely distributed local Indian population had a relatively balanced diet and an active outdoor life (Duffy 1979). Although these factors may have inhibited the indigenous development of the epidemic diseases that were the scourge of Western Europe, the North American Indians also seem to have been sustained by an elaborate form of traditional medicine that complemented other aspects of their lifestyle. This was based on a religion characterized by a Great Spirit ruling a number of lesser ones, in which it was thought that the slightest moral transgression could undermine the health of an individual. Within this belief system the medicine man played a crucial part by both invoking friendly spirits and warding off evil spirits. In these tasks, a range of devices were used – including botanicals, sucking, blowing and bloodletting. While there were superficial parallels with Western medicine, the primary distinguishing feature was undoubtedly the nature of the emphasis placed on the spirit world (Versluis 1993).

The main focus of this chapter, though, is on providing a backcloth to the rise of medical orthodoxy and the creation of the marginally defined practice of alternative medicine in Britain and the United States. This transformation can formally be dated from around the mid-nineteenth century onwards in the former and towards the end of the nineteenth century in the latter. To sketch in this background, the more detailed immediate historical context to the development of health care in the modern industrial world will be charted from the sixteenth century onwards. The analysis clearly demonstrates that, as in the case of their constitutional destinies, the trajectories of the two countries concerned were distinct, but not unrelated.

HEALTH CARE IN PRE-INDUSTRIAL BRITAIN

THE SIXTEENTH AND SEVENTEENTH CENTURIES

The most striking feature of the sixteenth and seventeenth centuries in pre-industrial Britain from the viewpoint of the interface between orthodox and unorthodox medicine is that health care was extremely varied in nature, with only a small minority of practitioners who could be regarded as officially sanctioned (Saks 1992a). Even more health care than today appears to have been undertaken on a self-help basis, with an appreciation of the value of a balanced constitution, and by other members of the public as a result of neighbourliness, religious duty and sheer necessity in the absence of resident practitioners. When health care was provided on a paid basis, moreover, it involved a wide range of health practitioners operating on a part- or full-time basis, often as itinerants. These spanned from female midwives licensed by a local bishop in testament to their character to empirics with little or no formal training (Porter 1995). It is argued that a plural healing system existed at this time, in which there was no clearly differentiated medical orthodoxy and no separately delineated sphere of alternative medicine (Stacey 1988).

This view is underlined by Larner (1992), who highlights the range of folk remedies available to individuals in Britain in the sixteenth and seventeenth centuries. These spanned from what she describes as ritual healing, involving charms and incantations, to practical medicine based on the use of plants and minerals. The remedies concerned included such practices as wearing amulets as a cure for colic, compilations of words to be recited to ward off suffering, cutting girdles on the sufferer to release disease, the use of ointments, and burning and burying animals and boiling the patient's urine with plant matter to drive out afflictions. The king was also endowed with magical powers as a healer as a result of beliefs in the divine nature of kingship – which helps to explain why the king's touch was widely used in the sixteenth and seventeenth centuries as a cure for conditions of the head, neck and eyes. It should not be forgotten, either, as Oakley (1992) points out, that women formed an important bedrock of grassroots health care provision. She particularly accentuates the significant part played by women healers in childbirth, a female role in health care which had roots going back to much earlier times (Duin and Sutcliffe 1992).

It is important to stress that there were also some 'official' practitioners at this time. Those with the highest status were undoubtedly the very small numbers of upper-class physicians educated in Greek medicine at universities in Britain and abroad. In serving élite groups, such as the royal family and the aristocracy, they depended heavily in their practice on expelling toxic substances through the traditional methods of purging, sweating, vomiting and bloodletting to restore the equilibrium of the body – in addition to using simple herbal preparations and complex compounded drugs from Arab and other medical traditions. This said, they tended to be very responsive to the wishes of their paying upper-class patients, who often took little heed of their advice (Porter 1995). Although their contemporary critics in Tudor and Stuart times were less than convinced of their worth against the ravages of disease, they achieved a limited monopoly in 1518 when they were incorporated by Henry VIII to oversee medical practice within 7 miles of the City of London, under the auspices of the Royal College of Physicians of London (Stevens 1966). This body was later complemented by the foundation of the Royal College of Physicians of Ireland and the Royal College of Physicians of Edinburgh in 1654 and 1681 respectively. Each acted on an independent basis, but had the common power to license physicians and oversee apothecaries within its sphere of jurisdiction.

The apothecaries to whom reference is made stood at the lower end of the spectrum in the emerging 'official' medical status hierarchy. Originally they were general shopkeepers who pursued a trade. However, they developed a distinct identity as part of 'official' medicine when they broke away from the grocers at the beginning of the seventeenth century to form the Worshipful Society of Apothecaries in 1617 – even if the training for their work remained underpinned by the apprenticeship as opposed to the university education of the physicians (Porter 1995). Although they initially simply dispensed prescriptions while the physician prescribed, operating under the authority of the Royal College of Physicians, they eventually won the right to treat the sick themselves following the exodus of the physicians and their wealthy patients from London during the Great Plague in 1665, becoming known simply as the Society of Apothecaries from 1684 onwards (Berlant 1975). This right to treat the sick was upheld early in the next century by the House of Lords. It enabled apothecaries to minister even more directly to the needs of patients. These were largely drawn from less affluent groups, inside and outside London – including in the provinces, where there were fewer restrictions on practice (Stevens 1966).

The other part of 'official' medicine comprised the surgeons, who – as we have seen – practised a long-established craft going back beyond the sixteenth century. The two guilds that formally laid down the rules for apprenticeships were established in England as early as the fourteenth century. These were the Company of Barbers, whose members engaged in minor surgery, including bloodletting and the extraction of teeth, and the higher-status Guild of Surgeons, which was involved in such activities as manipulating dislocations, setting bones and performing amputations. They came together in 1540 as the Company of Barber-Surgeons, which was to persist until the eighteenth century (Cule 1997). Its practitioners were usually required to serve a seven-year indentured apprenticeship. They primarily practised external medicine, rather than internal surgery, as the latter was too dangerous and painful before the introduction of anaesthetics and antiseptic techniques (Porter 1995). Socially, they stood between the apothecaries and the physicians in the pecking order in sixteenth- and seventeenth-century British medicine. Their strongest affinity, though, was probably with the apothecaries, who, together with the surgeons, increasingly acted as general practitioners for the lower classes and those living outside the major towns and cities as the eighteenth century approached (Stevens 1966).

Larner (1992) notes that the Witchcraft Acts reinforced the position of these three types of medical practitioner in relation to the various exponents of folk medicine in Britain. These Acts were employed against those who claimed to possess special powers not sanctified by the Church in the sixteenth and seventeenth centuries. Such powers were frequently alleged to have been used, among other things, to cast magical spells to bring about fevers, swoonings and swellings, sometimes with fatal consequences. The Acts seem to have been particularly used against female midwife-healers. The background to their implementation, according to Oakley (1992), was that such practitioners challenged hierarchical authority at a number of levels – including that based on religion, class and gender. In the latter respect, the enforcement of the Acts came at a time when male members of the developing medical bodies were closing ranks in a patriarchal society in which women were being increasingly discredited and disadvantaged, not least in the growing university sector.

However, it was still far too early to see this as signifying the practical achievement of a dominant medical orthodoxy, not least because of the relatively small numbers of licensed practitioners, the barriers to access to them, the limitations of their educational base, their general lack of corporate power, and the apparent lack of effectiveness of their remedies in fighting illness and disease in a religiously based society only too aware of its own mortality (Porter 1995). Most importantly, its position was limited by the difficulties which the fragmented medical authorities had in effectively enforcing the limited restrictions that existed in relation to both insiders and outsiders, even at a local level (Saks 1995b). That orthodox medicine in Britain at this time could not be clearly differentiated from the practice of other healers is well illustrated by the case of astrology. As Wright (1992) observes, while the belief that individual health is affected by the configuration of the planets may be regarded as marginal in most Western health systems today, astrology still underpinned the practice of élite members of the Royal College of Physicians, including one of its presidents. Thus in the seventeenth century there was a continuing overlap between the knowledge employed by folk practitioners and that used by medical practitioners of the day.

THE EIGHTEENTH CENTURY

If medical practitioners had not distinctly attained the higher ground of medical orthodoxy in the sixteenth and sevententh centuries in Britain – enabling the ready identification of alternative medicine – the same was still true by the end of the eighteenth century. Changes occurred over the ensuing hundred years, but the ground had not shifted to the extent that writers such as Maple (1992) would have us believe. He describes this period as the 'great age of quackery', in which a host of ignorant and avaricious 'quack' practitioners of a range of preposterous treatments are contrasted with upstanding regular medical practitioners striving to protect the public, under the banner of science. While this may have reflected the invective of many 'regular' practitioners at the time, the picture was by no means as clear-cut. As Porter (2001: 12) states, the boundaries were blurred and contested in an age in which there were 'individual medical practitioners of many stripes, some more, some less, engaged in quackish activities'.

That said, it would be foolish to ignore the development of 'official' medicine in this period. This can be illustrated by the work of major European figures such as Morgagni and Auenbrugger on relating disease to internal anatomical organs and on percussion diagnosis respectively (Cule 1997). Their work provided a significant context to the growing influence of the three bodies representing the Royal College of Physicians that Stevens (1966) documents, from a primarily local, metropolitan base to the whole of the country with which each of the separate colleges was associated. As she notes, surgery also moved forward in the latter part of the eighteenth century with the work of pioneers such as Hunter, the founder of surgical pathology, and the general refinement of surgical techniques. Linked to this progress was the new framework in which surgery came to be organized in Britain following the separation of the surgeons from the barbers. This involved the incorporation of the Royal College of Surgeons of Edinburgh in 1778, the Royal College of Surgeons of Ireland in 1784, and the Royal College of Surgeons of London in 1800.

The apothecaries too, according to Stevens (1966), built on the House of Lords ruling that had consolidated their position early in the eighteenth century, in the face of opposition from the Royal College of Physicians of London. In so doing, they gradually developed their role from running chemists' shops to compounding prescriptions and treating patients in their own homes. The change was complemented by the emergence of voluntary hospitals in the eighteenth century, in which the physician made all major medical decisions, working with the lower-status surgeons. The physician and surgeons together provided guidance to the resident apothecaries undertaking the tasks of bleeding, cupping and blistering. The voluntary hospitals themselves were founded as charitable institutions for the sick poor, serving as a training ground for the private care of the wealthy at home under their physicians. The less affluent meanwhile were dealt with as outpatients through the newly established dispensaries (Porter 1995). In such a system there was clearly a commitment to developing medical knowledge. In medicine the Enlightenment is epitomized by the decline in the eighteenth century of medical practitioners' subscription to astrology (Wright 1992). On the surface at least, this decline would seem to belie claims about the lack of distinction between 'official' and 'unofficial' practitioners.

In addressing the claims made about 'quackery' among unofficial healers in the eighteenth century, moreover, Porter (1994) clearly accepts that many still operated with little or no training, often using self-styled titles such as 'professor'. As he himself describes, there were also those who swindled patients, like the huckstering mountebanks with their monkeys satirized in plays of the period and those who published false testimonials and health warnings about not following the treatment offered in newspaper advertisements. Such swindlers particularly affected the more marginal and vulnerable groups in society, from the impotent to the infirm. It is difficult to believe that harm was not caused, given that the cures variously prescribed included such remedies as the inhalation of nitrous oxide for consumption, which was offered at the end of the century at the Beddoes' Pneumatic Institute in Bristol. Such 'unofficial' practitioners may also have served to divert patients from other, more appropriate treatment through their sweeping panacea claims, as exemplified by the hype surrounding Ward's pill, which was seen as a cure-all, and Graham's electromagnetic Celestial Bed for treating impotence and infertility. Neither could be fully justified in terms of the available evidence.

However, against this, the frailties of the 'irregulars' may have more to do with the ostentatious non-medical practitioners who were striving to displace physicians, than with the comparatively restrained rank and file. The latter relied largely on local handbills for publicity and restricted their activity to providing simple cures for such conditions as ruptures and toothache (Barry 1987). It would also be naive to ignore the limits of 'official' medicine itself in eighteenth-century Britain. Aside from the pain and other perils of the heroic measures practised at the time, doctors in the eighteenth century were not beyond excesses – such as dangerously administering over-large doses of mercury for venereal disease (Bynum 1987). Furthermore, as Porter (1994) notes, the public expected more of 'official' medicine than it was able to deliver, as, with the development of a more 'scientific' frame of reference, it began to become increasingly distant from the patient. The new approach emphasized the observation of symptoms, rather than the explanation of sickness. It was in part because of this, he claims, that the public was persuaded to shop around and consult with 'irregular' practitioners as it felt necessary.

The potential benefits of health care outside the practice domain of the physicians, surgeons and apothecaries should also not be ignored – including that of wise women, who were legally excluded from the developing medical corporations. Porter (1994) provides a helpful corrective to conventional wisdom by arguing that the reasons why those labelled as 'quacks' proved so popular in the eighteenth century cannot simply be explained by the fact that the gullible public had been duped. He believes that their treatments probably met a range of needs and did no more or less harm than those of 'official' practitioners. Indeed, he notes that many of those regarded as 'quacks' in the eighteenth century were the forerunners of currently extolled specialists, focusing on particular conditions such as those of the ear, eye and throat. They were practising, moreover, at a time when anyone other than a generalist tended to be decried. From another perspective, the numerous ready-to-use medications and guides provided by the 'irregulars', from Culpeper's *Herbal* onwards, undoubtedly facilitated the continuation of a self-help tradition. This remained of central importance in health care, reflected in the preventive emphasis placed by individuals on such methods as cold-water bathing and vegetarianism to strengthen their constitution (Porter 1995).

It was not simply 'irregular' practitioners who were involved in the entrepreneurial culture of the eighteenth-century marketplace, a culture that was responding to the high sickness rates and associated consumer demand in the developing capitalist economy at this time. As Porter (2001) observes, even the foremost practitioners of 'official' medicine were willing to cash in on patent medicines and proprietary pills with secret formulae. In Georgian times, making money out of nostrums and self-publicizing activities was seen by doctors as good business. Only in the Victorian era did professional ethics begin to be taken more seriously. The same was equally true of surgery. Barry (1987) suggests that 'regular' practitioners publicized operations on conditions such as cancerous breasts and cataracts through papers and pamphlets, in order to advance their careers. This, after all, was an age in which paying patients dominated in a predominantly fee-for-service system where even élite physicians had to be responsive in manner and style of approach to their affluent paying clients (Jewson 1974). To balance matters out, the so-called 'quacks' generally appeared as keen as medical practitioners to display their wares in the shop window of charitable practice, in line with the mainstream social values of the day.

The parallels do not end here. Porter (1994) notes, in relation to claims about the avariciousness of the 'irregulars', that doctors in the eighteenth century – while later distancing themselves from the more mercenary aspects of the marketplace – were as happy as their competitors to accept large fees. Their willingness to do so did not prevent the medical élite from joining the cultural circles of the fashionable high society of the day (Porter 1995). Nor was it only 'unofficial' medicine that relied on magic, sideshows and sleight of hand. Porter (1994) claims that such practices mirrored the ritual use of Latin mumbo-jumbo and the occult wisdom of humours and urine analysis in more 'official' forms of medicine. On the other side of the equation, those outside 'regular' medicine in the eighteenth century often also seemed to be seeking to steal its prestigious scientific thunder by justifying their approach with reference to such figures of medical reverence as Hippocrates and Galen. It should not be too surprising, therefore, that there was much overlap between the content of the practice of 'official' and 'unofficial' health care at this time. The two appear to have shared more similarities than differences.

Stevens (1966) argues that the same certainly was the case in relation to the 'regular' practice of physicians, surgeons and the apothecaries in the eighteenth century, these becoming increasingly difficult to distinguish, especially with the emergence of the general practitioner. Such a pattern was perhaps to be expected when the practical basis of their training had so much in common. While only physicians and some surgeons had degrees from British or Continental universities, what bound the three branches of medicine together was their use of apprenticeship training. This seems to have persisted because vocational rather than university arbitration of standards was established early in the development of medicine in Britain. The result was that medical schools were founded by practising doctors, with staffing in the growing numbers of hospitals being centred on bedside instruction to medical students. This form of training broadly mirrored the apprenticeship system by which many 'irregular' practitioners traditionally learned their trade (Stacey 1988), a system based on overlapping knowledge in which, among other things, the remedies prescribed were very similar in terms of active ingredients (Porter 1995). Taken together with the continuing difficulties of legally enforcing boundary demarcations (Saks 1995b), the similarity in training helps to explain why the orthodox/unorthodox interface still remained relatively fluid and undefined by the end of the century.

It is worth commenting on why the so-called 'quack' should have been so denigrated as a dangerous outsider consumed with greed over the course of the eighteenth century by those associated with 'official' medicine. In this context, occupational power and self-interests are undoubtedly central concepts in the rivalry that arose. Porter (2001), though, warns against assuming that the invective against the 'quack' in the eighteenth century was simply a manifestation of the move of doctors to professionalize, as in the first half of the nineteenth century. He argues that viewing it in this way involves stripping the events of that era from their pre-modern historical context, in which medicine is best seen as more of an occupation than a professionalizing vocation. For him, the war of words is best viewed as deriving politically from the developing marketplace associated with the growth of the middle classes and industrial capitalism, in which medicine was commodified and practitioners of all types

> were competing for custom, recognition and reward. Each in his own way – top physician, humble general practitioner, empiric, folk healer – made his bid to seize the moral high ground in a medical arena in which the law was acknowledged to be dog-eat-dog. (Porter 2001: 30)

This competitive environment helps to explain other, related developments in health care in eighteenth-century Britain. These include the ousting of female midwives by male accoucheurs or obstetricians in providing services for the well off. Midwifery proved too tempting an opportunity for market capture, notwithstanding the efforts of the 'man-midwife' to pass off the takeover as being related to the ignorance and incompetence of the traditional 'granny midwife' (Donnison 1977). In this regard, it should be underlined that nursing as we know it today had not yet strongly emerged as a force in the marketplace, although it did have an evolving role in the developing hospital sector. Given the limited apparent effectiveness of medicine at this time, nursing outside domestic situations – where women in the household and domestic servants played a key part (Stacey 1988) – was mainly linked to religious orders ministering to the spiritual needs of patients (Dingwall *et al.* 1988). However, the competitive market framework was becoming increasingly important. This also applied in the parallel case of health care in the immediate pre-industrial era in the United States, where it was no less easy to distinguish a clear medical orthodoxy.

HEALTH CARE IN THE PRE-INDUSTRIAL UNITED STATES

THE SIXTEENTH AND SEVENTEENTH CENTURIES

As noted earlier, health care in North America in the sixteenth century was based primarily on the elaborate tradition of Native American medicine. This was linked to its spirit philosophy and emphasis on healing through such means as the use of poultices and massage – complemented by the use of splints for fractures and clean water to wash out wounds (Duffy 1979). A range of botanical drugs were also used in their crude form by Indian tribes, including emetics to induce sweating and diuretics to increase urination (Rothstein 1988). It should be stressed, though, that, while grounded in similar principles, the North American native traditions at this time were diverse (see Taylor 1995). In the area that is now the United States, the nomadic Plains tribes predominated – from the Sioux and the Pawnee to the Crow and the Dakota tribes. They variously drew on sacramental and shamanic southern and northern traditions. Within this framework, the medicine man was a central figure in health and healing, relying on incantations, chants, dances, amulets and other forms of magic (Versluis 1993). This role was derived from that of the shaman, a religious figure involved in calling spirits to assist in healing tribal people. Either men or women were able to enact the role and usually obtained their position through some form of apprenticeship (Wilson 1997).

Believing that the source of illness lay in the supernatural world, the medicine man would perform magic not only to bring rain and enhance the fertility of fields, but also to cure fevers and expel the spirits thought to have taken possession of the bodies of the sick. In this latter case, as Kingston (1976) relates, the ceremony might involve the elaborately garbed medicine man dressed in the skin of a wild animal advancing on the sick person, leaping, shouting, waving his arms and shaking sticks or a rattle to frighten the demon in order to drive it out. Sometimes, pain was sucked out of the body through a tube of bone or hollow reed. Victims were given objects such as teeth and bright stones to wear, too, to protect against the evil eye – as well as talismans such as a rabbit's foot to give good fortune in the future. Soul catchers were also used by witch doctors to bring back the soul of the sick, as it was believed that sickness was caused when the soul was removed from the body by magic. Music and rhythmical movements, moreover, were held to create an appropriate atmosphere for healing to occur (Kaptchuk and Croucher 1986).

However, as Duffy (1979) highlights, the coming of the Europeans made an increasing impact on this healing culture from the sixteenth century onwards. It not only led to massive changes in the basis of North American health care, but also dramatically affected the health of the indigenous Indian population as it came into contact for the first time with diseases such as smallpox and tuberculosis. These seem to have been the main reason for the depopulation of New England in the early seventeenth century and the virtual elimination of the eastern Native Americans in colonial times. According to Duffy, for all the opportunities that the New World opened up, the new settlers initially had high mortality rates in the harsh conditions that they encountered there, after the dangerous ocean journey to America. Of the nine thousand new arrivals in Virginia, only just over one thousand remained by 1625. However, although Native American medicine was enthusiastically used by the early pioneers, and America was affected by beliefs in witchcraft (Starr 1982), it was the broader European – and especially British – form of health care that came to dominate as the Indian population declined and the settlers took ever stronger root.

Stevens (1971) nonetheless describes the development of medicine itself, which coexisted with the native traditions, as 'slow and uncertain' from the seventeenth century onwards. The slowness was largely the result of the scientific and cultural lag between Europe and America. She notes that the few medical practitioners in the separate colonies such as New England that rapidly developed were mainly ship's surgeons, apothecaries and those who had acquired medical skill by other means in Europe. They undertook a role similar to that of the surgeon-apothecary in the provinces in England, as opposed to that of the physician or barber-surgeon. Stevens argues that the colonies could not afford the luxury of the three branches of medicine that developed on the other side of the Atlantic, as these were socially rather than functionally grounded. Nor, in terms of political ideology, were they keen to replicate the hierarchies involved. The picture that emerged in the new settlements, therefore, was one of medical unity, with all-round practitioners who dispensed their own drugs. This arrangement was reinforced by the fact that the harsh life in North America held few attractions for the university-trained European physician élite (Starr 1982).

One result of the relative lack of health care practitioners in the colonies was that a range of men in fields other than medicine – such as law and teaching – acted as doctors, as well as following their own calling. There was a particularly strong association in this respect between medicine and the ministry throughout the seventeenth century, as exemplified by the situation in Massachusetts, where many clergymen dealt with both the bodies and the souls of their patients (Berlant 1975). This helps to explain the stronger emphasis that Stevens (1971) notes was placed in the decentralized North American system on natural history and practical common sense in health care, linked to the botanical exploration of the New World. This included knowledge of the work of Culpeper on herbal treatments, which was as widely known as in Britain through the publication of popular texts (Gevitz 1992). It should also not be too surprising that the training of doctors was more heavily based on an apprenticeship and self-education model in a society where universities were yet to develop as widely as in Europe. Indeed, by the end of the seventeenth century there were still no medical schools, licensing laws or medical societies in existence to provide public control over standards, even though some colonies were beginning to establish guidelines for practice (Stevens 1971).

In these circumstances, there was clearly even less of a dividing line in the fragmented political structure of the colonies between orthodox and unorthodox health care than in Britain. Health care was even more of a populist phenomenon, with the family at the centre. In this respect, Rothstein (1988) notes that books of recipes of herbals were extensively drawn upon by the North American colonists, who used the raw materials as leaves or powders for consumption in everything from teas to snuff. In so doing, they were following in the tradition of the explorers of America from Columbus onwards, who had sought out apparently efficacious botanical medicines to take back to Europe – even if some of their remedies were also imported from across the Atlantic. In the colonial period most medicines seem to have been grown and manufactured in the household, owing to the cost and lack of availability of the imported alternative, particularly in rural areas. Unlike in Britain, proprietary medicines did not become widely accessible in shops until after the eighteenth century.

THE EIGHTEENTH CENTURY

That the dividing line between orthodoxy and unorthodoxy was still less than clear by the eighteenth century can be illustrated with reference to the midwives, who initially came with the first female settlers. Duffy (1979) notes that until the middle of that century, they dealt with virtually all work in obstetrics, calling a doctor only when there were difficulties, and also serving as nurses and paediatricians. Their work – mixed with that of caring for the new mother's family and widespread public self-help – seems to have been based mainly on folk knowledge. However, as compared to Britain, there appear to have been fewer empirics practising without any systematic knowledge. The more learned doctors had usually at least read medical textbooks. Like their counterparts in Britain, they tended to employ heroic treatments such as bloodletting, purging and bleeding, remedies based on balancing bodily equilibrium and enshrined in the ancient Galenic humoral theory. Surgery was usually employed only for such emergencies as fractures and tooth extraction. The generic term 'physician' increasingly came to be ascribed to this group and to other self-defined doctors.

Such eclecticism persisted in the eighteenth century. In this period there were far more physicians than today in the United States, because of the lack of medical licensing regulation. According to Stevens (1971), they also began to open their own apothecary shops, as engaging in the pharmaceutical business by selling preparations made up by their apprentices was often necessary for them to survive (Rothstein 1988). Importantly, in terms of the competitive market in which such physicians increasingly operated, they successfully continued to oppose efforts by Americans trained in Britain to establish the tripartite British medical structure in the North America of the eighteenth century. A structure of that kind was not welcomed in the anti-monopolistic cultural milieu of the colonies – especially since it also militated against the interests of the mass of rank-and-file practitioners. The main difference that informally developed by the end of the eighteenth century was between those trained through apprenticeships and those educated in the growing university sector in Europe and North America. In this latter respect, a number of indigenous medical schools were formed, such as at the University of Pennsylvania in 1765 (Bynum 1994). Indeed, by the time of the Revolutionary War of Independence, which concluded in the early 1780s, several local medical societies were also in operation and an increasing range of states had medical licensing arrangements (Starr 1982).

Thus there was a growing distinction in the eighteenth century between a relatively amorphous group of 'regulars' and 'irregulars', paralleling that in Britain. Those in the former category typically had a longer training, limited codes of ethics and more established practice networks – and were becoming more unified in so far as they tended by now to practise medicine, surgery, pharmacy and midwifery (Stevens 1971). The 'irregulars', on the other hand, as Duffy (1979) notes, were operating more on the basis of pragmatic knowledge, often working part-time in isolated communities. They included native Indians, whose cures were often well regarded by the public, as well as other botanical practitioners, bonesetters and midwives – in a field that was still well populated by women (Starr 1982). 'Regulars' were represented at the high-status end by the more learned minister-physicians. These did not, though, always have the highest public profile. More famous were the likes of practitioners such as Perkins from Connecticut, who, having been expelled from his local medical society, propagated the use of magnetic tractors as a cure for all kinds of illnesses in the latter part of the century – building on work on animal magnetism by Mesmer (Gevitz 1988b). However, this is not the only reason why the dividing line between the two groups was blurred even as the end of the eighteenth century approached.

As in Britain, there may have been little difference in the effectiveness of the practice of the typically higher-class and male 'regulars' and that of the 'irregulars', as neither group in the eighteenth century could do much to prevent, cure or relieve disorders (Ehrenreich and English 1973). As Rothstein (1988: 34) notes, in a comment that is equally applicable to the British situation at the time:

> The existence of cells, bacteria, and viruses and the composition of blood and other bodily fluids were unknown; the functions of most organs were not well understood, and some had not yet been discovered; diagnostic tools like the stethoscope, X-ray, and ophthalmoscope had not been invented, and the thermometer was not yet used in medicine. Scientific knowledge existed only in gross anatomy, and it was of little value in daily medical practice. Theories of the causes of disease were based on such concepts as foul odors in the air and constriction and dilation of the blood vessels. Diseases were grouped into families based on superficial similarities, such as their symptoms or the part of the body affected. Descriptions of the natural history of diseases were unreliable because physicians unknowingly grouped different diseases having similar symptoms. Medical treatments were symptomatic and often actually harmful.

Although physicians did have some knowledge about the actions of drugs, the respect given to practitioners in the North American, as well as the British, context seems to have derived more from their personal characteristics than from their performance as doctors (Duffy 1979). The importance ascribed to personal characteristics was reflected in the individualism of much medical practice. Even in relation to pharmaceuticals, physicians prescribed a very broad range of preparations for similar conditions, based on a mixture of their own preference, the availability of the remedies and the tastes of their patients. The individualism of their practice was also grounded in the wide variety of their training, in which the idiosyncrasies of one generation of practitioners tended to be passed on to the next. The position was also further muddied by the relative absence of strong medical networks – either through medical societies, journals or proximity to other physicians in the rural communities in which they usually worked (Rothstein 1988). All this individual variation made it very difficult to distinguish 'regulars' from 'irregulars' in the developing United States context, in an age in which Duffy (1979) notes that medical theories were mostly practised without due regard for their implications for the patient. Ehrenreich and English (1973) in fact have argued that the 'regulars' may have been even more guilty of this, because of their stronger commitment to heroic interventions, as opposed to milder herbal and dietary treatments.

In terms of formal differentiation between orthodox and unorthodox practitioners, moreover, even the fragmentary licensing structures that began to develop did not significantly distinguish them. The statutes underpinning these – which also established ethical codes excluding professional relationships with outsiders – were generally ill defined, and rarely enforced where they did spring up, not least because juries would not normally convict the unlicensed (Duffy 1979). Indeed, responsibility was not even necessarily given to the relevant medical society as distinct from the government – as illustrated by the New Jersey licensing system established in 1772 (Berlant 1975). Attempts by medical societies to deny 'irregulars' consultations with 'regular' physicians and set up uniform fee schedules to discourage competition were not successful either; not only was membership of such societies low, but rules differentiating members from outsiders were frequently ignored. Efforts to distinguish 'regulars' from 'irregulars' on the basis of their graduate status were thwarted too by the sheer profusion, and lack of control of standards, of medical schools (Starr 1982); even though some schools attached to universities set reasonable benchmarks, their currency was diluted by the development of an increasing number of proprietary medical schools offering cheap, fast-track doctorates (Bynum 1994).

Defining the boundary line between the 'regulars' and the 'irregulars' in the United States was again further complicated by the fact that even the former group of physicians seem to have been prompted by competition with empirics to prescribe popular remedies (Duffy 1979). They did so doubtless in part because the earnings from medicine were not particularly high, although the fees charged by physicians were often felt by the public to be exorbitant (Gevitz 1988b). The issue of financial security affected even some of the most successful rural-based physicians in a fee-for-service system that was more starkly defined than in Britain. In the American colonies at this time there were no dispensaries, and charitable care for the sick was the exception rather than the rule. This position was offset only by the establishment of the occasional hospital or almshouse for the poor. Competitive self-interests in this entrepreneurial framework may also help to explain – as in Britain – why 'regular' physicians were so critical of the ignorance and lack of skill of the many so-called 'quacks', whom they saw as a danger to the public (Duffy 1979). This was a period when virtually anyone was able to practise healing; there was no shared body of knowledge and little legal restraint (Rothstein 1988).

We should not lose sight of the fact that, as Starr (1982) relates, most care of the sick still took place in the home by the end of the eighteenth century, as in Britain. Treatment was by now even more strongly based on naturalistic practices – although these were still underpinned by ideas about divine providence – with a parallel emphasis on factors such as diet and environment in prevention. Women typically dealt with any illnesses that arose, using herbal and other remedies that they kept to hand. Usually it was the wives who were pivotal here, working in the supportive context of the family and the community in which they lived. While the oral tradition remained crucial in the transfer of health knowledge, with publishing developments orally transmitted knowledge was increasingly complemented by the availability of a number of practical domestic health-care manuals, paralleling those that appeared in Britain. Importantly in this context, books like the widely selling *Domestic Medicine* by Buchan, published in 1769 and regularly reissued, were typically written in simple language and disparaged the extensive professionalization of health care (Gevitz 1992).

However, as in Britain, the situation was to change markedly in the nineteenth century – albeit in the United States in the second rather than the first half of that era. The seeds for further development in the United States lay in the period from the mid-eighteenth century onwards, in which Starr (1982) observes that a few educated doctors strove to enhance the professional standing of medicine. He notes, though, that while they succeeded in organizing medical schools and improved their status in face of their rivals, they initially 'failed in their larger effort to establish themselves as an exclusive and privileged profession' (Starr 1982: 30). That development did occur, though, as the nineteenth century progressed – first in Britain and then on the other side of the Atlantic.

THE PROFESSIONALIZATION OF MEDICINE IN THE NINETEENTH CENTURY

THE PROFESSIONALIZING PROCESS IN BRITAIN

Crucial to the more rapid move to professionalize medicine in nineteenth-century industrial Britain was the development of an increasingly unified medical community and the desire to raise the variable level of education and practice to a common baseline. Initially this took place in the face of resistance from the Fellows of the Royal College of Physicians in London, Edinburgh and Dublin. However, their strategy shifted in a more democratic world in the light of attacks by liberal philosophers and politicians striving to maximize economic competition in the marketplace, a world where it was no longer feasible for the physicians to claim sole legal rights to medical practice in their desire for monopolization (Berlant 1975). In this respect, there was no single standard of medical education at the beginning of the nineteenth century, with nineteen different bodies having the power to license practitioners (Parssinen 1979). Medical practitioners at this time were generally seen as distinctly marginal, with a thin line between doctors and shopkeepers, even among those regarded as the more respectable. As Parssinen (1979: 111) notes, their reputation was not enhanced by the fact that they also encompassed 'drunken, randy medical students; half-caste army and navy surgeons; impecunious Scots with dubious medical degrees in their kits; and irreligious professors of anatomy who furtively purchased exhumed corpses from graverobbers'.

However, the élitist Royal College of Physicians continued to advance its position – with its strong links to the Universities of Oxford and Cambridge in England and its emphasis on the value of an education in classics, morals and manners to provide the social polish to fit its members into high society (Bynum 1994). Despite its influence in government circles, though, its restrictiveness meant that by 1834 there were only 274 licentiates and 113 fellows as compared to the many thousands of apothecaries and surgeons (Stevens 1966). This meant that the practice of physicians was largely limited to ministering to the very rich in the biggest cities (Parssinen 1979). It is not surprising, therefore, that as the nineteenth century wore on, the Royal College of Physicians faced increasing competition from practitioners from the other two branches of medicine as consumer demand grew in the provinces and elsewhere. This challenge was amplified in the unfolding modern era in which its status credentials were diluted by the development of the newly emerging ethos of occupational professionalism, based on the certification of technical competence and the public service ideal (Elliott 1972). This dilution took place despite the fact that at this point the licence of the Royal College of Physicians remained exclusive and could not be held in conjunction with that of any of its medical rivals (Stevens 1966).

The surgeons formed an important part of this challenge. They began to attain a standing equal to that of the physicians by the start of the nineteenth century in Britain, as their craft grew into a more intellectual discipline, building on the establishment of the Royal College of Surgeons in 1800 (Waddington 1984). The rise of this Royal College was also fostered by the growth of medical education, in which each major hospital had developed its own medical school by the beginning of the nineteenth century, staffed by physicians and surgeons (Stevens 1966). But if this testifies to the growing professional status of surgeons, who like the physicians were increasingly taking up key consultancy roles in the hospital sector, it should be remembered that teaching in medical education was still subordinated to practice. Nonetheless, mainstream medical practice was beginning to shift from 'bedside' to 'hospital' medicine, based on the surgical legacy of Hunter and the proliferation of European advances in this field. The shift enabled growing stress to be placed on generic classificatory approaches to disease, as distinct from the more individualized person-centred medicine focused on the expectations of particular clients that preceded it (Jewson 1976).

By the start of the nineteenth century many apothecaries also acted as surgeons, as both of these groups sought to enhance their educational standards. A major breakthrough as regards the former was made with the passing of the Apothecaries Act in 1815. In spite of their continuing association with shopkeepers and their clear legal obligation to dispense the prescriptions of physicians – which attested to their subordinated status (Waddington 1984) – this gave apothecaries the right to examine and license in England and Wales. The requirements included attendance at lectures, six months' experience at a public hospital, infirmary or dispensary, and a five-year apprenticeship. The Act also enabled them to prosecute those in practice without a licence. The licence itself, together with membership of the Royal College of Surgeons, rapidly became the aim of most medical students being trained at recognized medical schools (Stevens 1966). The underpinning legislation mainly reflected reformist pressures from general practitioners in the provinces and helped to protect the 'regular' practitioners – by now the vast majority – from competition from the more lowly retail druggists, even if the latter were still not formally outlawed (Porter 1995).

It was this context that by the mid-nineteenth century in Britain provided fertile ground for the professionalization of medicine on a national basis and the formal creation of what is now regarded as orthodox medicine. Importantly, the three branches of the medical profession progressively came closer together, largely as a result of pressure from below. Indeed, these branches did not map directly on to everyday medical practice in the first half of the nineteenth century, as distinctions between them were increasingly blurred on the ground. Their amalgamation at a wider level was particularly facilitated by the development of peer-based journals such as the *Lancet* and the *Provincial Medical and Surgical Journal*, the latter of which was later to become the *British Medical Journal* (Bartrip 1990). The formation of the Provincial Medical and Surgical Association, the forerunner of the British Medical Association, in 1832 was also central to this process. The reforming provincial practitioners who constituted the rump of its membership had increasingly gained medical degrees and/or were licentiates of the Society of Apothecaries and members of the Royal College of Surgeons (Porter 1995). From the latter part of the 1830s onwards, they stepped up their petitioning of Parliament for legislation aimed at establishing a single medical organization, the standardization of medical education, and criminal sanctions against unlicensed practitioners (Parssinen 1979).

That said, what would shortly come to be defined as alternative medicine as a result of their success still had its appeal in the first half of the nineteenth century, as the lay population was increasingly able to purchase health care in the wake of industrialization. At the same time, as Porter (1995) relates, individualism, liberty, purity and self-help became ever more important to the self-improvement ideals of artisans and the labouring classes in the new capitalist industrial era. These led, among other things, to the wide use of various forms of herbalism, including that of the medical botanists of the Thomsonian school, imported from the United States in early Victorian times. They sought to free the poor from the prejudicial effects of the 'old school' of medicine by encouraging trust in nature (Gevitz 1988b). Homoeopathy too became extremely popular, especially with the aristocracy and wealthy clients from the emerging bourgeoisie – not least for its relative safety (Nicholls 1988). Other similar therapies, such as hydropathy (based on naturopathic water cure), also came into vogue by the mid-nineteenth century, as demand for them was buoyed by economic expansion (Brown 1987). These developments were paralleled by the mushrooming field of patent medicines as a wide array of ointments and pills flooded on to the market as the century progressed (Duin and Sutcliffe 1992).

Such competing therapies, nonetheless, were increasingly marginalized, as the Provincial Medical and Surgical Association and other bodies lobbied for medical registration in the public interest from the 1830s onwards. In the process, rival practitioners such as the hydropaths and homoeopaths were attacked as 'quacks' for harming patients, while stripping them of their money by charging excessive fees. Thus the *Lancet*, for example, depicted homoeopathy in this period as either a dream or a new preparation used by charlatans – and argued that it should die a death, given its own absurdity (Nicholls 1988). At the same time, the Royal Colleges were able to use their influence to prevent those linked to such therapies from entering their 'official' training posts, and thereby effected a degree of internal control over the nascent profession (Saks 1996). Those already firmly lodged within the ranks of medicine who practised therapies strongly associated with their competitors came under siege too. A good illustration is the case of Dr John Elliotson, an eminent professor of medicine at University College Hospital in London, who became involved in such practices as mesmerism, a popular cultural phenomenon of the day. He was forced to resign his chair in the latter part of the 1830s as a result of his 'irregular' activities (Parssinen 1979).

Such an adversarial stance could be seen, from a neo-Weberian perspective, as being in the group self-interests of medical practitioners in pursuing a monopolization strategy in face of competition. This particularly applies to the Royal College élite, but is also relevant to the broader constituency of doctors, many of whom were not financially secure, in powerful positions or of high social status at this time. It was certainly true of doctors working in the Poor Law services for sick paupers and for friendly societies and benefit clubs to which those in the lower orders of society subscribed. They often had little autonomy, a relatively low income and a large workload in the buyers' market that existed (Porter 1995). The efforts of medical practitioners to weaken the position of their rivals and engage in collective social mobility (Parry and Parry 1976) had hitherto been limited by such obstacles as the failure of juries to support action against those infringing their jurisdictions. The juries' attitude was understandable in view of the public support given to their competitors and the difficulties that the incipient profession had in enforcing internal control, given the wide span of licensing bodies and medical theories on offer (Saks 1996). However, by the mid-nineteenth century, the first unified national system of professional licensing in health care was established through the 1858 Medical Registration Act, which gave the new profession significantly more power.

The enactment of this legislation was not straightforward. It took seventeen different bills presented to the House of Commons between 1840 and 1858 before the Medical Registration Act was passed (Waddington 1984). That the delay occurred – despite the government's desire to establish statutory regulation of the medical profession – could be explained by the divisions between the different branches of medicine over the form that registration should take, as well as the contemporary state of medical knowledge. While a number of innovations had been introduced into medicine in the first half of the nineteenth century – such as the stethoscope, introduced by Laennec (Duffin 1999) – there was still a long way for it to go in terms of technical development and effectiveness (Dally 1997). The time for allied health occupations to become part of medical orthodoxy was also yet to come. It was only from the mid-nineteenth century onwards, for example, that Florence Nightingale instigated her campaign to reform nursing (Dingwall et al. 1988). The more developed formation and social closure of the nursing and midwifery professions lay over half a century ahead in the British context – almost as far away as the time when medical licensing was to be fully achieved in the United States.

THE PROFESSIONALIZING PROCESS IN THE UNITED STATES

Orthodox and alternative medicine thus became more clearly delineated by the mid-nineteenth century in Britain, even though exponents of the latter were still able to practise under the common law (Saks 1996). In the United States such a position seemed remote by the end of the first half of the nineteenth century. The initial signs immediately after the turn of the century were encouraging from the viewpoint of the medical monopolists, as physicians endeavoured to enhance standards and establish professional regulation (Stevens 1971) in a manner designed to develop a group rather than an individual identity (Marcus 1996). As a result, there was a proliferation of medical societies, medical schools expanded and licensing began to take off – even if the licences that were issued had variable provisions (Berlant 1975). However, these moves were challenged as public opposition to the creation of licensing monopolies grew as a result of the very openness of American society itself. Such opposition was exemplified in Ohio and Illinois, where the state legislatures had initially empowered medical societies to issue licences in 1811 and 1817 respectively. Here licensing was never rigorously enforced, and was subsequently rescinded in the period from the late 1820s to the early 1830s – as it was in such states as Mississippi in 1836, South Carolina, Maryland and Vermont in 1838, Georgia in 1839 and New York in 1844 (Starr 1982).

Starr (1982) argues that this shift occurred mainly because physicians had to ride the storm of Jacksonian America in the 1830s and 1840s, in which their claims to privilege were rejected on the basis of the prevailing anti-corporatist philosophy. Berlant (1975) places more emphasis in explaining the change on the popularity of their competitors and the difficulty of justifying medical society licensing as a touchstone of competence at this time. The outcome, though, was the same – namely, that arguments that the 'scientific rationalism' of physicians should supplant 'quackery' were overridden by a preference for free competition over monopoly. It was left to members of the public themselves to be the arbiters of their own health care, at a time when those employing herbs and other folk remedies were flourishing on the basis of their inalienable right to practise medicine. As in Britain, allowing the public to come to their own decisions was consistent with democracy – albeit in a system in which differences in medical rank were considered inappropriate and greater faith was placed in the public itself. In this political culture, as the capitalist economy developed in the Jacksonian era, people were held to have free and equal rights to judgement in face of the potential emergence of professional monopolization. As Porter (1992: 8) observes, in the United States in this period the 'knowledge ethic was aggressively democratic, anti-corporatist, and individualistic'.

The existence of this socio-political environment meant that physicians seeking to create an élite profession – with boundaries against competitors established through licensing and professional societies – were always likely to be rebuffed. As Starr (1982) notes, the political climate supported unrestrained competition among health workers, in which those who defined themselves exclusively as physicians encountered market pressures to reduce the cost and duration of their training. Physicians certainly faced intense competition from practitioners such as the Thomsonians, who were formed into 'friendly botanic societies' and aimed to progress the interests of 'ordinary men' at the expense of their authority. The Thomsonians coexisted, among others, with homoeopaths, hydropaths and the sellers of a wide variety of nostrums (Gevitz 1988b) – not to mention Native American medicine men (Duffy 1979), who also rivalled physicians. Self-help was encouraged too by the publication of more guides to domestic medicine, which were particularly used by women in the home (Gevitz 1992). Although few of these were by North American authors, the ones that were employed tended to treat their readers as equals, draw heavily on anecdotes and avoid much of the technical terminology so common in guides published in Britain. They can clearly be seen as part of the popular health movement which peaked in the 1830s and 1840s (Ehrenreich and English 1973) – in which Grahamism was central in propagating the benefits of everything from vegetable diets and hygiene to abstinence and exercise (Whorton 1988).

It remained difficult to differentiate orthodox and alternative medicine in other ways at this stage. In part, it was difficult because, in the face of sectarian competition and consumer demand, 'regular' practitioners moderated their more excessive heroic therapeutic practices (Rothstein 1972). As Starr (1982) relates too, some remedies employed by 'regular' physicians, such as quinine, were also used by 'irregulars' who drew on their learned authority. Moreover, while the practice of folk therapies by women probably decreased as the century wore on – as the role of midwives and other female healers declined with the increasing acceptance of the claim of 'regular' physicians to superior skills – the number of females in 'regular' medical practice grew. In this regard, women increasingly began to enter medical education after the mid-nineteenth century, despite continued ostracization by the medical societies. The relative lack of differentiation between 'regular' and 'irregular' practitioners was reinforced by the fact that only a minority of physicians were educated in medical schools and their therapies were still of questionable effectiveness – as highlighted by the therapeutic divisions within medicine itself. This was despite technical advances in medicine, the growing replacement of traditional practices by modern, empirically-based clinical methods and the limited, self-taught knowledge employed by many 'irregulars' at this time.

The relative lack of differentiation between orthodox and alternative medicine before the American Civil War may well have contributed to delays in the introduction of medical professionalization in comparison with Britain. It was accentuated by the more market-based economy of the United States, where government investment in health at federal and state levels was even more sharply limited to such provision as facilities for mental illness and contagious diseases (Stevens 1971). This restrictiveness – together with competition from both rivals and colleagues in an overcrowded private sector in which it is estimated that there were around seven thousand 'irregular' practitioners and sixty thousand physicians by the mid-nineteenth century (Berlant 1975) – meant that there was relatively low usage of medical services. Usage was also constrained by the limited buying power of consumers and high travel costs in rural areas, which left many physicians in a precarious financial position. Their difficulties were compounded, in the largely credit-based, fee-for-service health system in which they operated, by the relative slowness of the development of general hospitals as compared with Europe. As a result, a large number of physicians had to keep on another job for a living, perhaps working as a farmer or drug store proprietor (Starr 1982), further blurring the boundaries with their competitors.

This context helps to explain the uncomfortable group relationships between some 'regulars' and 'irregulars' at this time. If we leave aside the invectives of Thomsonians about the abolition of the authority of doctors, lawyers and other such groups, exclusionary strategies, as Warner (1987) points out, tended to be more directed by the former at the latter. Unlike in Britain, groups such as the homoeopaths had a self-identity of already being members of the 'medical profession'; they were seeking to reform more aggressive allopathic practices from within. Even so, they variously accused the 'regulars' of being 'mercury dosers' engaged in 'murderous systems' of 'humbuggery practice'. However, in response, physicians spoke of 'rational effort' being 'paralysed by medical scepticism' and a reliance on nature by charlatans 'destroying' the patient. At a wider level, physicians also distanced themselves from the sectarians by excluding them from the medical societies that helped to socialize members into patterns of conformity, as well as barring them from 'regular' medical schools. The situation of both the 'regulars' and the 'irregulars', though, was to change with growing professionalization in the United States over the next half-century, albeit in ways that reflected its own distinctive national political structure.

This change, as in Britain, was not straightforward, given the major conflicts between rival schools of physicians that increasingly broke out from the mid-nineteenth century onwards. Starr (1982) notes that these divisions in a competitive environment formed the largest obstacle to the collective medical social mobility that had occurred in Britain. Such divisions were deep, and in evidence at all levels, from professors in medical schools to more humble local medical practitioners, notwithstanding the unifying effects on the group identity of physicians of growing local medical society membership and developments in clinical medicine. Rifts were fostered by the emergence of societies and associations in fields such as ophthalmology, neurology, dermatology and surgery, as growing numbers of physicians saw it as in their interests to define themselves primarily as specialists, as opposed to general practitioners (Stevens 1971). This was a time, moreover, when the social position of physicians – whether operating in the private, public or the expanding charity sector – was highly variable and based more on their family connections, education and the standing of their patients than on membership of the medical community *per se* (Starr 1982).

In the next half-century, though, the overall income, status and power of doctors rose in line with what had been achieved earlier in Britain. Crucial to this shift was the founding of the American Medical Association in 1847, shortly before the establishment of the American Pharmaceutical Association in 1852. This body, initially centred mainly on younger, less established physicians, strove to introduce ethical barriers to professional relationships with outsiders (Stevens 1971). It also sought to increase and standardize medical educational requirements, assisted by visits to prestigious European medical schools (Bynum 1994). That the Association was not immediately successful in achieving its aims was mainly because, in the absence of widespread licensing, it lacked authority over its members at a time when political infighting was rife in a relatively open field (Krause 1996). However, its activities did help to keep out 'irregulars' from federal medical office and make it more difficult for 'regular' practitioners to step outside defined occupational boundaries. The Association also provided a more unified platform for gaining the licensure underpinning the professionalization of medicine in the early twentieth century. This professionalization was facilitated, among other things, by the founding of medical periodicals such as the *Journal of the American Medical Association* and an expansion in the number of general hospitals, which progressively lost their lower-status tag as treatment outside the home increased. Stronger corporate interests thereby developed, as the social distance between patient and practitioner grew (Starr 1982).

External competitors were still in existence at this stage in the United States. Their survival was encouraged by the continuing use of heroic therapy by many physicians, which included practices such as bleeding and purging that were increasingly falling out of public favour (Rothstein 1972). Porter (1994) refers to the burgeoning numbers of 'toadstool millionaires' who sold patent medicines in the latter part of the nineteenth century. These were hawked along with devices such as ozone generators for a range of conditions that included malarial fever and diphtheria, often with an absolute guarantee to cure these and other ills. He notes too the growth of spiritualism based on female faith healers as the nineteenth century progressed, together with the development of Christian Science through Mary Baker Eddy (see Schoepflin 1988). These tendencies complemented the popular health reform movements that were also a defining feature of the second half of the nineteenth century, centred on books by such key figures as John Harvey Kellogg (O'Connor 2000). Britain and the United States shared an open free-trade position in relation to 'irregular' practitioners, as compared with the tighter official regulation that was imposed to curb their spread in many other Western countries in this period. In this context, the American Medical Association – like its British counterpart – was virtually powerless to stop their practice in the Victorian era (Starr 1982).

Thus we see that the distinction between orthodox and unorthodox medicine had not fully emerged in the United States even by the latter half of the nineteenth century. In fact, as Thomsonism declined, further competition came from a number of other major medical sects – including principally the homoeopaths and the eclectics, who built on most of the tenets of Thomsonism without denying the need for scientific training (Gevitz 1988b). Both these sects – which were themselves striving for professional standing – established a range of colleges from the 1850s onwards and began to challenge physicians on the grounds that greater rather than lesser complexity was required in medicine. However, they in turn continued to be systematically attacked by 'regular' physicians, who often strove to minimize professional contact, paralleling the antipathy towards such practitioners in Britain. At a macro level, the American Medical Association reinforced the position by placing strong pressure on state medical societies to exclude sectarian practitioners (Burrow 1963). Such actions, though, did not prevent the numbers of eclectic and homoeopathic schools growing to 22, as compared with 76 'regular' schools by 1880, with the 'irregulars' accounting for around 20 per cent of the total number of medical practitioners (Starr 1982).

Ironically, however, as Starr (1982) points out, this growth was to provide the common ground that was to accelerate the cause of medical professionalization in the United States. One of the distinctive features of the United States in the late nineteenth century was that although the eclectics and the homoeopaths were split over the merits of associating with physicians, they saw it as in their interests to work with them to gain licensure, and thereby protect themselves from untrained competitors. There were, of course, divisions within the ranks of 'regular' medicine itself about the acceptability of such accommodations, notwithstanding the stringent line taken by the American Medical Association on this issue. Rank-and-file physicians had a number of incentives to cooperate: they had failed to gain effective licensing restrictions over their rivals on their own; they already had widespread informal linkages with the 'irregulars' in practice; they feared the impact on their incomes of open warfare; and some of the more extreme philosophies of the sects concerned were being abandoned. The motivation to collaborate may also have been increased by the growth of specialization based on developing medical knowledge at the end of the nineteenth century (Stevens 1971). This had the effect of increasing the interdependence of the homoeopaths, the eclectics and the 'regulars' in terms of referrals and access to key facilities (Starr 1982).

The result of such cooperation was to establish a network of state licensing boards, dominated wholly or partly by state medical societies, across the United States (Berlant 1975). As Starr (1982) notes, the establishment of these boards took place in a changing socio-political context in which the growth of major industrial corporations had transformed professional licensing from being a disdained privilege of the powerful, as it was in the first half of the nineteenth century. Instead, in the latter part of the century it became an important part of the defence of their trading rights with individual consumers in the face of competitors. The licensing regulations that gradually emerged in individual states were at first typically based on a minimum requirement of diploma-level education, with the caveat that long-established practitioners could continue to operate. The regulations were then extended, as in Illinois in 1877, where all physicians had to register and diplomas from inappropriate schools were rejected, putting thousands of practitioners out of business. The main resistance to such licensing predictably came not so much from the 'irregulars' – who had either separate boards or representation on the main boards that were established – as from those who did not meet the standards adopted. The courts, however, generally upheld such state licensing arrangements, and they became increasingly widespread. Associated with such arrangements was the upgrading of medical education – of which the hospital-based Johns Hopkins Medical School came to be regarded as a model, following its foundation in the 1890s (Krause 1996).

The consequence for the eclectics and the homoeopaths was that they became incorporated into the mainstream. Their practitioners and independent schools were rapidly absorbed after the turn of the century (Rothstein 1988; Kaufman 1988). New areas of marginal practice were thereby created, not least being that of the osteopaths, whose schools, associations and hospitals developed autonomously (Stevens 1971). By the early 1900s, therefore, the state had finally shifted its position, from indifference to physicians' claims to monopoly to accepting them as legitimate practitioners. At the same time, by 1905 the American Medical Association had reorganized the vast majority of its state and local medical associations on a uniform federal basis – leading to a considerable growth in its membership as local medical societies gained in strength (Starr 1982). A framework for the professionalization of medical orthodoxy was thereby created by the beginning of the twentieth century in the United States which – while different in its detail – nonetheless paralleled the British system that came into existence in the mid-nineteenth century. Although registration for nurses and other allied orthodox health professions occurred only later in the twentieth century in the United States (Duffy 1979), lines of demarcation were for the first time nationally established between orthodox and alternative medicine, as in Britain.

CHAPTER 2

The rise of the medical profession and orthodox biomedicine

This chapter focuses on orthodox medicine as it developed in Britain and the United States up to the mid-twentieth century, building on the historical background set out in Chapter 1. It starts off by describing in more detail the shape that the pivotal professionalization of medicine took on both sides of the Atlantic, and its wider significance. The chapter then considers some of the main theories as to why the medical profession should have gained the legally enshrined monopolistic position underpinning its ascendancy in the Anglo-American context. Finally, it examines the subsequent development of medicine up to the end of the first half of the twentieth century in both Britain and the United States. This includes the growth of orthodox biomedicine itself under the banner of 'scientific' progress, the expansion of medical specialization and the emergence of a range of allied health professions. Reference will be made where appropriate to the links to the field of alternative medicine created by the establishment and consolidation of medical orthodoxy. Alternative medicine, though, will be the primary focus of attention in Chapter 3, where an analysis will be given of the interest-based interplay between insiders and outsiders in the marketplace in the period up to the 1950s, based on the neo-Weberian approach on which this book is centred.

It is necessary initially in this chapter, however, to outline the nature and form that the professionalization of medicine took in the two main countries considered here. Before doing so, it should be emphasized that the legal regulation underpinning the associated process of social exclusion – which for the first time opened up a formally defined sphere of alternative medicine – represented a watershed in the division of labour in general and in the health care arena in particular. State regulation in the Anglo-American context has since been introduced in many other occupational areas and has come to cover a range of facets of professional activity, from policing market entry to controlling competing practices (Moran and Wood 1993). The form that such regulation has taken has varied greatly both within and between societies, even in the case of specific professions. In the health field, it ranges from more fully developed patterns of exclusionary social closure in medicine to more limited market shelters in other allied health professions. It is therefore important to explore the contours that closure took in the medical field in the mid-nineteenth century in Britain and the early twentieth century in the United States, especially given the central focus of this book on professionalization and health care.

THE CONTOURS OF MEDICAL PROFESSIONALIZATION IN BRITAIN AND THE UNITED STATES

MEDICAL PROFESSIONALIZATION IN BRITAIN

In Britain the 1858 Registration Act gave medicine a unique niche in the health arena which Parry and Parry (1977) see as representing a classic case of upward collective social mobility. It signalled the rise of apothecaries and surgeons – alongside the more prestigious physicians – to fully fledged professional standing. In this regard, many years of parliamentary campaigning resulted in legislation underpinning the claims of doctors for exclusionary closure. This legislation was centred on a system of self-regulation relatively free from lay control, in which a formal community of equals restricted recruitment through the maintenance of a register and the control of education and training. Thus the medical profession was granted a form of state monopoly in providing services in the marketplace, at the heart of which lay the General Medical Council (see Stacey 1992). This enhanced its position in terms of income, status and power, and proved an ingenious compromise from which all parts of the 'regular' profession gained benefit – including members of the Royal College of Physicians and Surgeons, as well as the Society of Apothecaries (Porter 1995). It is not surprising, therefore, that Waddington (1984: 96) has termed the Act 'a major legislative landmark – perhaps the major legislative landmark – in the development of the medical profession'.

As Waddington (1984) notes in outlining the detail of the legislation, its main thrust was to establish the General Medical Council, with the requirement that it maintain a register of all qualified practitioners. Importantly, this shifted the traditional mechanisms for regulating the newly formed medical profession from a local to a national level. In so doing, it weakened, but did not break down, the traditional divisions within medicine – emphasizing the unity of what was shared between its different branches. This unity was perhaps most apparent in the common codes of ethics that were adopted, for which aberrant registered practitioners could be disciplined through the central power of the General Medical Council. Importantly, too, the Act gave legal meaning to the notion of 'qualified medical practitioners' based on minimum standards and training – differentiating them from unqualified outsiders whose names were not on the official register. In this sense, the Act fulfilled the desire of doctors to restrict entry into what was perceived to be an overcrowded profession. However, it did not in principle exclude outsiders from practising, as they were still entitled to operate under the common law as long as they did not represent themselves as medical practitioners (Saks 1992a). This has remained the case even though, as we shall see, a number of pieces of legislation in the period up to the mid-twentieth century were introduced to restrict this entitlement (Larkin 1995).

Berlant (1975) has undertaken a detailed analysis of the formation of the British medical profession from the viewpoint of monopolization. He makes a number of key points about the 1858 Act. One of these is that in terms of the rights of doctors and, indeed, those who were henceforth defined as lying outside of the profession – such as lay homoeopaths and herbalists – this was a *de facto* as opposed to a *de jure* monopoly. It did not formally preclude the unqualified from practising. Nonetheless, it had the effect of bringing about a monopoly, because it put such practitioners at a considerable competitive disadvantage in the growing public sector and the private market. They were certainly disadvantaged in relation to their exclusion from government medical service, their inability to certify statutory documents, their exclusion from the legal right to recover medical charges and the lack of the state legitimacy that doctors gained as a result of being on the register. A further significant point that he makes is that the legislation was directed not only against outsiders, but also towards the diminishing competition that came from inside the profession, through the codes of ethics that were established in the general interests of its members. To complete the circle, these codes of ethics were additionally designed to restrict collaboration with non-qualified practitioners, for the medically qualified were at risk of being struck off if they infringed such provisions (Saks 1996).

MEDICAL PROFESSIONALIZATION IN THE UNITED STATES

As we saw earlier, in the United States the professional monopoly that arose came later, in a context of competitive individualism in which the majority of physicians remained self-employed in the private sector (Starr 1982). When the exclusionary closure of the profession emerged on a wide scale at the beginning of the twentieth century, it also differed in structure. One difference was that it was based on more fragmentary pluralistic political arrangements, with specific legislation governing the operation of physicians in each state rather than being cast on a national basis. By contrast, in Britain a more unified system developed with the 1858 Act, and, despite relatively minor variations in the organization of professional services across the national boundaries of England, Wales and Scotland (see Levitt *et al.* 1995), the divisions that increasingly emerged were more reflective of interprofessional differences than of geographically defined jurisdictions (Brazier *et al.* 1993). While a few professional groups have since come to be licensed by the federal government in the United States (Freidson 1986), the regulation of the medical profession in America set the standard for the growing ranks of other professions. These have subsequently also been subject to differential state licensing arrangements.

As Berlant (1975) relates, therefore, the establishment of increasing numbers of state boards by the start of the twentieth century was at the core of the professional regulatory system that emerged in medicine in the United States. These provided exclusive licences to practise medicine. A majority of each board, moreover, was typically made up of medical society representatives, which indicates the extent to which physicians themselves controlled the processes concerned. At the same time, the accreditation level of medical schools was raised for licensing purposes and to meet medical education laws defining the form of training that was required. While physicians could not stop outsiders from practising legally if − like the osteopaths and chiropractors − they had gained separate state licences in their own field, their rivals in the health care arena were still at a competitive disadvantage. Even if they won licensing rights, they were not normally able to gain access to hospitals and the right to prescribe drugs, which diluted the challenge to medical practice very considerably (Starr 1982). Thus the professional exclusion that emerged in the United States in the first years of the twentieth century could be seen as based more on a *de jure* than on a *de facto* monopoly along the lines established in Britain (Berlant 1975).

That said, despite differences in specific state licensing arrangements for medicine in the United States, there were a large number of similarities across the states in the regulatory arrangements established for American medicine. This was so even compared to most of the other professions that were to develop over the first decades of the century. By the start of the twentieth century, the high degree of cross-state patterns of regulatory resemblance in medicine was facilitated by the fact that licensing arrangements in most states were characterized by widespread domination by doctors, with local medical élites represented on relevant state boards (Moran and Wood 1993). In addition, the newly founded profession was seeking to upgrade general standards, which resulted in a more restricted membership of the medical profession nationally, given limits on the number of schools that met the stipulated criteria. The publication of the Flexner Report in 1910 on conditions in medical schools was a very significant factor in virtually halving their number in the period from 1904 to 1928. This was because such schools depended for their existence on recognition of their diplomas by state licensing boards (Berlant 1975). The national frame of reference in which this exercise was conducted highlights the fact that parochial licensing arrangements in individual states in this field were more limited than first meets the eye.

This point is underlined by the national role played by the American Medical Association. This body backed the Flexner Report, in so far as it had established the Council on Medical Education in 1904 to evaluate existing training in medical schools and had instigated the inquiry that was to follow. The American Medical Association's ratings of medical schools were accepted for accreditation purposes too by the Federation of State Medical Boards when they were published. These came to have the force of law, and encouraged increasing uniformity in the medical curriculum (Starr 1982). The Association also endeavoured to ensure consistency in other ways. For example, it issued a model plan in 1910 in relation to the organization of state and county medical societies, following an exponential rise in its membership from 1900 onwards. While medical domination over state societies has been restricted largely to minimizing interstate competition, a national perspective remained (Berlant 1975). The distance between licensing arrangements in Britain and the United States, therefore, may not be as great as imagined in terms of coherence – and indeed actual effect – even if there are still some differences in the detailed licensing provision between states.

Finally, it is important to note another parallel between the cases of Britain and the United States. As Larson (1977) says, the drive to professionalize medicine and other areas in the United States was also a collective mobility project that enhanced the socio-economic standing of those involved, as illustrated by the benefits of the subsequent market restrictions on physician supply that were facilitated by the Flexner reforms (Starr 1982). There was a major struggle before medical interests finally prevailed in the United States, just as in Britain – where it will be recalled that legislative attempts to formalize the professional standing of medicine were the subject of much protracted debate leading up to their implementation. In the American case, there was even resistance to local state medical monopolies, given existing anti-trust legislation and the antipathy of the general public towards monopolies. In Massachusetts during the 1890s, for instance, the National Constitutional Liberty League of Boston attacked medical monopolization on the grounds that it constrained the liberty of both the patient and the physician (Berlant 1975). Such attacks raise the question of why the British and

American medical professions were successful in effecting their own particular brands of exclusionary closure in the mid-nineteenth and early twentieth centuries respectively.

THEORIES OF THE PROFESSIONALIZATION OF MEDICINE

THE FUNCTIONALIST ACCOUNT

How then can the achievement of the various forms of professionalization in medicine underwritten by the state that led to the differentiation of orthodox and alternative medicine in Britain and the United States best be explained? Functionalist writers on the professions who held sway in the social sciences up to the 1960s – alongside their trait counterparts – usually tend to see this as part of a natural history of professionalization. They view it as being based on distinct sequential stages of development, including the establishment of training schools, the formation of professional associations and the adoption of formal codes of conduct (see, for instance, Wilensky 1964). From this vantage point, functionalist theorists generally regard the emergence of professions as being driven by occupationally based expertise of great value to society in the meritocracies that developed in Western industrial countries. This involves a trade-off in which the occupation concerned agrees to regulate its members through ethical codes and other means in the public interest in return for state-protected autonomy and associated privileges. The establishment of professions from a functionalist perspective is thereby held to meet the changing needs of the modern world (see, for example, Goode 1960; Barber 1963).

The functionalist view is well exemplified in the health arena by Wallis and Morley (1976). They specifically ask why medical pluralism in Britain and the United States should have been supplanted by the creation of consensual occupational monopolies of treatment in the Anglo-American context in the latter half of the nineteenth and early twentieth centuries. Wallis and Morley (1976: 11) argue that the monopolies related to the industrial revolution, which 'rapidly transformed both the demand for effective medical treatment and the ability of the profession to provide it'. Demand for treatment grew in part because the geographical and social mobility associated with urbanization broke down traditional ideas previously linked to the stable communities in which people lived, at the same time as expectations were heightened by the acceptance of basic citizenship rights in emerging meritocracies. Alongside this there was the development of science and technology, including the bacteriological revolution of the nineteenth century, which brought with it the germ theory of disease. It is claimed that in this situation, the professionalization of medicine arose to cope with disease and protect a vulnerable public from exploitation through registers of appropriately qualified medical practitioners who themselves controlled admission to the profession.

This slick functionalist argument, however, rests on a number of questionable assumptions, including the extent of social fragmentation that was associated with the industrial revolution and the ascription of the changes that did occur to industrialization and urbanization as opposed to the rise of capitalism (Saunders 1986). The most vulnerable aspect of this explanation, though, is that the rise of professionalization based on exclusionary closure was linked to the increased effectiveness of scientific medicine in providing remedies for illness at the time at which it was achieved. This seems particularly implausible in the mid-nineteenth century in Britain. Wallis and Morley (1976) claim too that the scientific rationalism of medicine ultimately overcame the more pronounced anti-intellectualism of *laissez-faire* American society in the early twentieth century, despite its history of tolerance of medical sects. This related explanation of medical professionalization and the creation of a sphere of marginal medicine in the United States unfortunately does not stand up strongly to critical scrutiny either. Rather, as in the British case, it appears more like a retrospective rationalization of developments in the medical arena.

In Britain the 1858 Medical Registration Act was passed long before the pharmacological revolution and other major advances in diagnosis and treatment in Western medicine which occurred well into the next century (Dally 1997). Moreover, heroic therapies based on bleeding and purging were still widely used by British doctors in the nineteenth century. The therapies employed by their competitors, such as the homoeopaths, also had their own merits – not least being their relative safety in comparison with some of the more extreme interventions of the 'regular' profession (Nicholls 1988). And while there was a growing awareness of anaesthesia and aseptic techniques in British medicine, these were still not generally employed by doctors in surgical operations and elsewhere before the passing of the 1858 Act. It is not perhaps surprising in this light that hospitals were popularly seen at that time as 'gateways to death' (Youngson 1979). It may nonetheless be more plausible to argue that scientific development underpinned the professional monopoly created in medicine across the various states in America some half a century later.

In this respect, Stevens (1971) certainly differentiates the United States from Britain in her detailed historical account in terms of the appropriateness of the timescale for justifying professionalization based on technical expertise. As the analysis of American medicine by Starr (1982) suggests, the state of medical knowledge in the second half of the nineteenth century in the United States was also limited. He comments that at this time, American medicine knew its limitations, without having the means to advance beyond these. However, even by the turn of the century the argument that the exclusionary closure of the medical profession could be explained with reference to its effectiveness is not ultimately compelling. As Berlant (1975: 236) says:

> The most productive advances in medicine were not to come until the twentieth century. The scientific method, in fact, had not entered American medicine until the 1860s. Orthodox medicine was still very much in a period of therapeutic nihilism, engaged in examining traditional practices with controlled studies for evidence of efficacy, at the time when the medical licensing laws were passed. The competence of the medical profession was not very convincing, even in the eyes of contemporary legislators; many states of the period passed licensing legislation which permitted irregular practitioners to practice, as long as they could pass a qualifying examination.

MARXIST EXPLANATIONS

If the professionalization of medicine in Britain and the United States cannot necessarily be justified by the adequacy of the scientific knowledge at the time at which the relevant legislation was enacted, perhaps it may be better seen as a socio-political creation dependent largely on conflictual relationships of power. In this respect, Marxist writers such as Navarro (1976, 1978, 1986) argue that the class relations of capitalism have been the main forces shaping the historical development of health provision in Britain and the United States. He claims that the medical profession in Britain and the United States emerged as part of the bourgeoisie, as capitalism developed. On this interpretation, it is suggested that the establishment of the privileged position of medicine cannot be appropriately understood if the profession is seen as autonomous. Rather, it needs to be viewed as an element of the ruling class contributing to capital accumulation by dealing with the disease and diswelfare associated with life under advanced capitalism.

This type of account, however, also runs into difficulties. While Navarro is by no means insensitive to the counter-productive effects of modern medicine, it is dangerous to imply that medicine was equipped to be effective in contributing to capital accumulation when it became a profession in Britain and the United States. He also underplays the complexity of the relationship between the medical profession and capitalism. This complexity is highlighted by empirical studies of the subsequent operation of the medical profession on both sides of the Atlantic, which indicate that it has not simply played the narrowly class-constrained role that Navarro perceives (see, for instance, Eckstein 1960; Starr 1982). Other writers within the Marxist camp more fully recognize the intricacies of the relationship. McKinlay (1977: 467), for example, acknowledges that physicians probably have some independent control of the medical game, even if 'the amount of control that physicians exert may actually be quite limited when viewed in relation to ... industrial and financial forces'. There are significant theoretical difficulties too from a Marxist perspective in including the medical profession as part of the ruling class, given that its members are not necessarily owners of the means of production. This forms part of the debate as to where the middle class may best be located in the Marxist analysis of the class structure (see Parkin 1979).

Johnson (1977, 1980) avoids this problem in his more focused and sophisticated Marxist-inspired account of why some occupations rather than others gain professional standing in the class structure. Drawing on the work of Carchedi, he sees professions as agents of capital in the labour process, not as members of the capitalist class, in a structure where there are divisions in the middle class itself. In theorizing the conditions under which professiona-lization strategies are successful, he distinguishes the global functions of capital associated with a small, high-status group and those of the collective labourer that involve tasks that are subject to routinization. Johnson (1977: 106) claims that the professional form of occupational control can emerge only 'where core work activities fulfil the global functions of capital with respect to control and surveillance, including the specific function of the reproduction of labour power'. In the case of medicine, he argues that this control is fulfilled by the role of doctors, who, through legislative means, monopolize official definitions of health and are able to define and legitimate the withdrawal of labour.

Nonetheless, such an approach again faces problems in explaining the origin of the professionalization of medicine. For all its theoretical elegance, relatively little is said about the distinctive elements of the control and surveillance function in which professions in general and the medical profession in particular are held to be engaged (Saks 1983). In a related manner, Johnson also fails to analyse systematically the functions of a comparative range of professions and occupations to evaluate the extent to which the theory stands up empirically. Such an analysis is needed, given that comparative research into the professions suggests that the process of gaining professional privileges is not straightforward. It may, for example, reflect structures and ideologies from previous historical periods as well as that of capitalism itself, as illustrated by the professional standing of the clergy (Portwood and Fielding 1981). Moreover, Johnson's argument is tautological, as it is based on a structuralist view of the state that is seen as invariably serving the needs of capitalist production (Saks 1987).

This element of tautology is also apparent in the latest contribution by Johnson (1995), which otherwise represents a clear departure from a Marxist approach. In this work, Johnson endeavours to apply Foucault's notion of governmentality to the politics of professionalization, including that of medicine. His analysis is centred on seeing the state and the professions as inextricably connected, rather than as diametrically counterposed. This position importantly stands against the received wisdom of much of the Anglo-American literature on the professions which posits that the state and the professions are separate, with the former seeking to extend its control and the latter aiming to protect and, where possible, enhance the autonomy of members. Following the conception of the modern state by Foucault as an ensemble of components that together define a particular form of government, Johnson contends that professional groups are themselves part of state formation and that professions such as medicine are the institutionalized form of expertise within this formation. This contention recognizes that the link between professional authority and the state is based on more than the power of professional bodies and includes many diffuse aspects of the work of professionals bounded by state regulation (Esquith 1987). Interesting as this notion is, however, similar problems of operationalization arise in health and other contexts in explaining the dynamics of professionalization if the boundaries between the state and professions are obscured in this way.

THE NEO-WEBERIAN APPROACH

The strongest applied contribution that Johnson makes to the analysis of the reasons why medicine gained a professional monopoly in Britain and the United States by the early twentieth century is contained in his initial work derived from a neo-Weberian frame of reference, on which this book is centred. Here Johnson (1972) argues, *inter alia*, that professionalism – based on the occupational authority of the producer over the consumer – as opposed to other forms of institutional control, is most likely to come into being where consumers form a large, heterogeneous group. He observes that this form of control emerged in medicine by the second half of the nineteenth century in Britain with the development of industrialization and the associated growth of an urban middle class. This enlarged middle class provided an expanding market for medical services and broke the bonds of upper-class patronage. He notes too that professionalism in medicine and other areas was facilitated by the creation of a more homogeneous occupational community which, among other things, increased the bargaining power of doctors. He also stresses that fostering upper-class recruitment to medicine to increase its standing furthered the process of professionalization. Upper-class recruitment is held to have complemented the development of links with powerful élites, which were traditionally very close between the higher-status members of the Royal College of Physicians and their aristocratic clientele in Britain.

This analysis fits well within a neo-Weberian perspective, which, as we have seen, emphasizes interest-based occupational strategies aimed at gaining control of the market through the establishment of exclusionary closure in a more pluralistically conceived social order. Some of the elements cited by Johnson as being involved in effecting social closure in medicine in Britain clearly also apply to the United States in the early twentieth century. They include such factors as the fragmentation of the clientele and higher-class recruitment to medicine (Starr 1982). There is some resonance in this respect with the work of Freidson (1970), who has analysed the medical profession in the United States from a neo-Weberian perspective, albeit with a definition of professionalism related to occupational control over the organization of work (Freidson 1994). He gives a number of reasons why the medical profession secured its privileged position in American society. These include the fact that medicine made itself attractive to the public and gained lay support for professionalization. He also emphasizes that it was vital for medicine to win state sanction for its claims, the state being the ultimate source of power and authority in society. Like Johnson too, he notes that it was crucial for the medical profession to gain the sponsorship of strategic élites by persuading them that there was special value in its work.

Berlant (1975) applies the Weberian concept of monopolization to medicine in both Britain and the United States, and therefore has additional comparative relevance in the present context. Using this framework, he claims that the success of organized medicine resulted from its tactics of competition as well as the socio-political conditions in the societies concerned. Importantly, he identifies some significant differences between Britain and the United States. He notes that the British medical profession in the nineteenth century successfully advanced its position through ideological reform to combat attacks by liberals on corporate monopolies. Its success in this respect is illustrated by the internal controls over the performance of professional practitioners by the General Medical Council that were accepted under the terms of the 1858 Act, in part because they did not preclude unregistered practice in the market. At the same time, he highlights how the American medical profession, like other professions in the United States, improved its standing by exploiting the political conflict between national and local economic interests in the face of the anti-trust movement. In this regard, the desire to protect local economic interests against the encroachment of national corporations and bureaucratization by encouraging local monopolies is seen to have helped to promote the widespread development of state licensing in medicine.

This is not to say that either this or other neo-Weberian analyses are flawless. Berlant, for instance, does not give sufficient emphasis to the socio-political context as opposed to the profession's ideological strategy in his analysis of the British case (Saks 1983). Freidson similarly provides too little empirical detail of the general factors he sketches out as underlying the professionalization of American medicine. This is exemplified by his lack of specificity about the nature of the strategic élites involved in the United States (McKinlay 1977). Johnson, meanwhile, in his neo-Weberian mode, is prone to making extravagant statements without fully recognizing the need for empirical evidence. This is illustrated by his unsubstantiated claims about the lack of technical skills of general practitioners in Britain not just in the nineteenth century, but in the twentieth century too (Johnson 1972). All the aforementioned accounts are also vulnerable to the charge of being gender-blind. They understate the importance of the fact that the profession of medicine was male-dominated in the patriarchal Anglo-American context, in which its professionalization claims succeeded in the latter half of the nineteenth and the early twentieth centuries (Witz 1992). The work of neo-Weberians to date, however, undoubtedly helps us to understand the reasons for the initial professionalization of medicine in Britain and the United States, which is pivotal to the underlying themes of this volume.

Having considered the viability of a variety of different theories of the professionalization of medicine, the discussion has so far been primarily focused on the form of professional regulation as it emerged a century or more ago in the Anglo-American setting. The nature of professional closure in specific occupational fields, however, can change over time in particular societies (Collins 1990). In this respect, current professions may be strengthened or weakened depending on factors ranging from wider technological and socio-political developments to the emergence of new professional groupings. As such changes occur, the privileges of professional occupations may ebb and flow – nowhere more dramatically illustrated on a wider canvas in the medical field than by the disenfranchisement of physicians with the emergence of Soviet-style socialism in Russia in the first part of the twentieth century (Field 2000). This is an appropriate juncture at which to examine the development of medical orthodoxy in Britain and the United

States in the period up to the 1950s, which – while generally going from strength to strength – took distinctive pathways on different sides of the Atlantic. Such an examination will provide a crucial context for considering the relationship with unorthodox medicine up to the middle of the twentieth century in the next chapter.

THE DEVELOPMENT OF ORTHODOX MEDICINE IN BRITAIN UP TO THE MID-TWENTIETH CENTURY

THE CONSOLIDATION OF THE BRITISH MEDICAL PROFESSION

As already indicated, the 1858 Act was only the first step in the professional regulatory process in medicine in Britain. Further reform occurred over the course of the next century. As Waddington (1984) observes, the 1886 Medical Act embellished its provisions by requiring all future candidates for entry to the profession to be examined in medicine, surgery and midwifery. This requirement reinforced the standardization of the qualifications of doctors under General Medical Council control – consolidating its role as the keystone of the new system of professional self-regulation. Waddington notes too that the effect of the 1858 Act was to restrict the growth in the numbers of medical practitioners over the next twenty years. Although these subsequently increased, he adds that even by 1911 there were still fewer medical practitioners in relation to the population than at the time of the passage of the Act. While this drop in numbers was related to the tightening up of the standards of medicine on a national basis under the General Medical Council, from a neo-Weberian perspective it also improved the market position of doctors – as in the Flexner period in the United States. As such, the restriction on numbers qualifying contributed to the generally enhanced prosperity of medical practitioners in Britain, even if pockets of financial deprivation continued to exist until the beginning of the twentieth century among those who worked in poorer areas (Stacey 1988).

The year 1911 was a watershed in medicine, as it marked the passing of the National Health Insurance Act. This provided for limited access to non-hospitalized medical care from general practitioners for workers covered by the legislation, paid on a capitation basis by wage deductions and contributions from the state and employer (Jones 1994). This arrangement largely supplanted the previous fee-based general practitioner system and was complemented by a patchwork of health insurance through friendly societies, trade unions and commercial firms. Importantly, aside from limiting class inequalities, it helped to reduce the growing rift between general practitioners and hospital specialists, as the hospital sector gained in popularity (Stevens 1966). It also provided some protection from alternative therapists and other unqualified competitors, as it confined the delivery of this extended provision to general practitioners (Parry and Parry 1976). The 1911 Act was followed in the 1920s and 1930s by attempts to extend health insurance and to organize medical services in a more planned way, in the face of inequalities in the distribution of general practitioner services and the continuing expansion of hospital care. These efforts ultimately culminated in the 1946 National Health Service Act, which was the next major landmark in terms of national health provision and was not without significance for the market position of doctors in Britain (Allsop 1995a).

The 1946 National Health Service Act led to the founding of the National Health Service in 1948, building on the Beveridge Report, which is commonly regarded as a blueprint for the modern welfare state. While the private sector continued to exist, this legislation provided for a more comprehensive state service free at the point of delivery, based on capitation payments for general practitioners and a salaried hospital service (Kingdom 1996). Such state intervention in health has frequently been seen in the United States as the epitome of 'socialized medicine', imposing excessive bureaucratic constraints on doctors – ultimately leading to their deprofessionalization (Elston 1991). It is certainly true that members of the British medical profession put up considerable opposition to the National Health Service initially, in part because of their fears of losing their autonomy (Allsop 1995a). However, as Berlant (1975) points out, the state financing of health care in Britain in practice increased the income, status and power of the medical profession because of the enhanced market advantages that it offered from a monopolistic interest position. Although hospital consultants probably benefited most from its implementation, general practitioners also retained their independence and consolidated their standing (Gill 1975). Significantly, too, the National Health Service Act helped the profession as a whole to further marginalize its rivals, as alternative practitioners were legally excluded from the state medical service (Saks 1994).

The development of orthodox medicine in Britain from the mid-nineteenth to the mid-twentieth century, though, cannot be understood in abstraction from the self-conscious links fostered with 'science' that helped to legitimate its position, following the Enlightenment. As Waddington (1984: 198) notes,

> although the increasingly scientific basis of medical practice [in the aftermath of the 1858 Medical Registration Act in Britain] had no immediate or dramatic impact in terms of therapeutic effectiveness, nevertheless the cultural status of science almost certainly lent prestige

and authority to medical men, and may well have been a significant process in increasing the level of demand for their services.

Nor was the kudos of 'science' just window dressing in relation to the developing medical orthodoxy, for it also gave rise to the growing promise of therapeutic success as the twentieth century unfolded. Contributors such as Brandt and Gardner (2000) describe the decades either side of the turn of the twentieth century as the 'golden age of medicine', as fundamental changes took place to transform and make more systematic medical knowledge, practice and policy. This systematization process led to an increasingly unified and consensual body of theory, based on biomedicine, around which medicine henceforth became centred (Saks 1995b). Crucially, this ideological orientation towards 'scientific' biomedicine enabled the medical profession to differentiate itself from its non-medically qualified alternative practitioner rivals.

The development of biomedicine was based mainly on a modernist conception of the body as a symptom-bearing organism, with drug and surgical intervention to the fore (Saks 1998a). It should not be assumed, however, that biomedicine is rooted in a static body of knowledge. Its capacity for change is highlighted by Jewson (1976), who noted the general transition that we saw in Chapter 1 from 'bedside' to 'hospital' medicine in the period from the eighteenth to the nineteenth century. This led to growing stress being placed on generic classificatory approaches to disease, as distinct from the more individualistic, person-centred medicine that preceded it. As he observes, orthodox medicine underwent a further fundamental metamorphosis with the development of 'laboratory' medicine by the first half of the twentieth century in Britain and other Western societies. In this framework, the patient became conceived as a cluster of cells – with micro-organisms increasingly being associated with specific diseases, as postulated by the germ theory of disease developed by Pasteur and Bernard in France in the nineteenth century. This new concept was linked in the British context, among other things, to the diagnosis of conditions such as anaemia through the microscopic examination of blood cells, public health reform, and enhanced surgical procedures in the latter half of the nineteenth century. These were variously followed by the growing use of radiotherapy to treat cancer cells from the early years of the twentieth century, and the employment of antibiotics in the treatment of infectious diseases from the mid-1930s onwards (Dally 1997).

For all their potentially beneficial effects, though, such changes to the nature of orthodox medicine, based on the notion of 'scientific progress' in Britain and other industrial societies, are seen by Jewson (1976) as depersonalizing and disempowering for the patient. This is not surprising in an era when it was felt to be increasingly possible to diagnose diseases through the analysis of samples by technicians who had never personally met, and were often physically far removed from, the patient. The distance so created was also increased by the growing marginalization of the subjective opinion of the client in the period up to the mid-twentieth century, as a result of the intensified laboratory focus of orthodox biomedicine. In this regard, the positivistic biomedical approach contrasted with earlier, pre-industrial approaches to health care involving the interplay of mind and body – as well as some of the more holistic contemporary practices of their rivals in alternative medicine, such as homoeopaths (Nicholls 1988). The resulting disjuncture can be traced back to the classic division that Descartes, the French philosopher, made between mind and body in the seventeenth century – which undoubtedly had a major formative influence on Western medicine (Saks 1997a).

The disempowerment of the patient in the century following the 1858 Act, however, conversely gave greater strength to the profession itself – based on the growing technological expertise underpinning biomedicine. This was particularly true as far as hospital specialists were concerned, for such roles provided opportunities for making scientific reputations to enhance their eminence and authority (Porter 1995). According to Waddington (1984), increased specialization was also in part linked to the growing market for medical services that sustained full-time practice in niche areas. Although the concept of specialism had earlier been tainted by its association with 'quack' rivals and was regarded by general practitioners as threatening to their interests, Britain witnessed the growth of a wide range of medical specialties, from obstetrics and gynaecology to ophthalmology and paediatrics, by the mid-twentieth century. Indeed, even in the nineteenth century, as knowledge of particular areas increased, close to one hundred specialist hospitals were founded in London alone (Dally 1997). This trend was to accelerate in the first half of the twentieth century, albeit at the cost of degrading the general practitioner and further fragmenting the health care experience, from the viewpoint of the patient.

Such fragmentary influences on the profession were exacerbated by the growing rift between grassroots practitioners and the increasing numbers of full-time researchers associated with the new paradigm (Jewson 1976), as bodies such as the Medical Research Council entered the picture (Brandt and Gardner 2000). However, the development of 'scientific' biomedicine paradoxically led to greater uniformity of undergraduate medical education in Britain in the period under consideration. This was especially evident following the decline of the apprenticeship system in the second half of the nineteenth century (Waddington 1984). The result was a reduction in particularistic relationships in medical education and its increasing location in formal institutional contexts that encouraged the development of a common professional identity. This process was further facilitated by the emergence of national and regional centres that drew students from all parts of Britain, based on the values of leading figures in the profession. These centres increased the extent of monolithic professional socialization determined by a small medical élite drawn from the British Medical Association and the Royal Colleges, exercised through the General Medical Council. Professional socialization had the effect of not only further distancing students – the practitioners of the future – from the influence of the public, but also enhancing the power of the profession against outsiders. This power was augmented by the development of a referral system between specialists and general practitioners that increased professional solidarity among colleagues (Saks 1995b). That said, different requirements for specialist training in professional education at postgraduate level were established in this period (Stevens 1966).

THE EMERGENCE OF THE PROFESSIONS ALLIED TO MEDICINE IN BRITAIN

Further differentiation in the ranks of orthodox medicine in Britain up to the mid-twentieth century also resulted from the emergence of a series of professions allied to medicine, from pharmacy to nursing. The nature of the legislation underpinning such health professions provides a sharp contrast to that supporting the market position of the medical profession, which remained dominant in the increasingly elaborated division of labour. Turner (1995) categorizes the two main forms of professionalization for such allied medical practitioner groups as 'limitation', in which the operation of a professional group is restricted to a specific part of the body or therapeutic method, and 'subordination', in which a profession takes on tasks delegated from doctors. These are to be distinguished from his third category of relationship to orthodox medicine – that of 'exclusion', in which practitioners are denied formal registration altogether. Exclusion relates most closely to non-medically qualified alternative therapists, who will be considered in more detail in Chapter 3.

The category of 'limitation' best describes the emergence of pharmacists, dentists and opticians, who by the mid-twentieth century had together gained the most extensive pattern of social closure, outside of medicine, in the health sector in Britain (Saks 1998b). The Pharmacy Acts in the 1850s and 1860s permitted the Pharmaceutical Society of Great Britain to register pharmaceutical chemists, legally precluding the unqualified from dispensing medicines

(Levitt *et al.* 1995). The position of dentists was similarly underwritten by the 1878 Dentists Act, which allowed the General Medical Council to examine and register such practitioners. It was followed by legislation in the 1920s and 1930s providing for the formation of, first, a Dental Board and, subsequently, a General Dental Council (Nettleton 1992). Ophthalmic opticians meanwhile eventually established the General Optical Council in the 1950s to obtain the legal right to their autonomous professional territory in the health care marketplace (Larkin 1983). All these professions, however, gained their independence from direct medical supervision in the market at the expense of being trapped within their own narrowly defined jurisdictions – thus reinforcing the position of medical dominance won by doctors as a result of their own monopolization strategy in the mid-nineteenth century.

The establishment of professions based on the category of 'subordination' in this period is well illustrated in Britain by the case of nursing. This form of professionalization was based on the 1919 Nursing Registration Act, which founded the General Nursing Council as the regulatory body in this area (Rafferty 1996). The closure effected by this legislation was tempered by the fact that the place of nurses in the pecking order was determined by the existing monopoly of the medical profession over diagnosis and treatment. In this respect, nurses followed closely on the heels of the midwives, who had gained their subordinated professional market shelter through the Midwives Act of 1902. The position of midwifery was additionally circumscribed by the fact that the Board that was to regulate them had a medical majority and was not even required to include a midwife among its members. As Stacey (1988: 91) notes, this enabled the medical men of the nineteenth century

to create a new male-dominated gender order. They had the right of attending any birth; they had secured for themselves the right and responsibility of handling all difficulties and complications in childbirth and had made it the midwives' responsibility to see that they were called in such cases. They had ensured that the midwives would be trained in the way they thought right.

The cases of the professional subordination of nursing and midwifery in the first half of the twentieth century are by no means unique in the British context. The professions supplementary to medicine, with seven separate boards – for chiropodists, dietitians, medical laboratory technicians, occupational therapists, remedial gymnasts, radiographers and physiotherapists – were ultimately formed on a similar basis under the umbrella of the Council for the Professions Supplementary to Medicine in 1960 (Larkin 1983). It is easy to see why they – like the nurses and midwives, who gained a restricted form of exclusionary closure some half a century before – are often described as 'semi-professions'. Neo-Weberian contributors such as Parkin (1979), though, prefer to conceptualize their position as one of 'dual closure'. This is because, having failed to gain full professional closure, they are held to combine the exclusionary aspects of credentialism based on a register with the usurpationary tactics of organized labour. In this respect, there are similarities between the relationship of medicine to such professions and that of personnel such as nurses and midwives themselves to health care assistants and other kindred groups in the evolving health care division of labour in the first part of the twentieth century (Saks 1998b).

Before we shift our attention to the development of medical orthodoxy on the other side of the Atlantic in the period up to the 1950s, it should be noted that there are debates as to why such limited and subordinated groups should have gained this form of professional standing. These parallel those surrounding the professionalization of medicine, considered earlier. In the example of nursing, functionalists such as Etzioni (1969) argue that this is because such occupations need less expertise and training in fulfilling their role in the division of labour. Neo-Weberians, however, instead tend to link such outcomes to interest-based turf battles with medicine, centred on income, status and power, in which nurses were faced with a developing medical–Ministry alliance in late nineteenth- and early twentieth-century Britain (Larkin 1995). Abel-Smith (1960) indicates how nurses were able to advance their position through royal patronage and the precedent of registration set by the midwives in the 'thirty years war' that culminated in professional registration in 1919. However, they had to concede medical supremacy. What stood against their gaining the full exclusionary closure of doctors appears partly to have been the comparatively lower social class background of many of the nursing rank and file. A further crucial factor may well have been the conception of nursing as 'women's work' in a predominantly patriarchal society – in which nurses were competing against a profession that was heavily male dominated (Garmarnikow 1978).

This is an area, though, that is not uncontentious. Some neo-Weberian writers have put forward arguments about the position of such occupational groups in the Anglo-American context without adequate empirical support. An example is the unsubstantiated claim of Johnson (1972) that the historical subordination of the professions auxiliary to medicine in the health care division of labour in Britain, instigated by the medical profession through the state, was 'irrational'. There are also debates between Marxist and neo-Weberian contributors as to how far the role of the state in the subordination of women in the health professions is based on its operation as a capitalist state, rather than because it simply functions on patriarchal lines (see, for instance, Witz 1992). It is clear, however, that – notwithstanding the professional pecking order in health care – nurses and the other professions allied to medicine shared some of the benefits with doctors of the 1911 National Health Insurance Act and the introduction of the National Health Service in 1948. These enhanced the position of all the professional groups within medical orthodoxy in Britain, by reinforcing its *de facto* monopoly against outsiders, dominated by doctors. How, though, did the position of medical orthodoxy develop in the United States in the first half of the twentieth century?

THE DEVELOPMENT OF ORTHODOX MEDICINE IN THE UNITED STATES UP TO THE MID-TWENTIETH CENTURY

THE CONSOLIDATION OF THE AMERICAN MEDICAL PROFESSION

Following the building of the professional base in medicine in the United States by the start of the twentieth century, the next four or five decades saw a substantial consolidation of its power – which paralleled in different ways the British experience. This was by no means a straightforward process. Starr (1982) argues in his analysis of the period from 1900 to 1930 that there were a number of threats to the professional independence of medicine in the largely private, relatively uncoordinated health system that developed in the more *laissez-faire* American economic system. They included the growing establishment of corporations in health care, such as companies that employed physicians to provide medical care to workers and mutual benefit societies. These endangered the autonomy of physicians, as well as threatening to drive down the cost of medical services that detrimentally affected the fees they could charge. The rapid growth of the private hospital sector offered too a similar challenge, with the added threat of the rationalization of the individualized traditions of solo practice in an ever more hierarchical and bureaucratized context.

However, Starr (1982) notes that instead of succumbing to these challenges, by the 1920s the medical profession – which was increasingly well represented through the American Medical Association (Moran and Wood 1993) – had successfully enhanced its collective position compared to what it had been at the turn of the century. It did so by, among other things, moving on from long-standing sectarian quarrels, gaining stronger licensing laws, and establishing even greater control over the supply of physicians. In this process, such potential threats as the expanding hospital sector were turned into bulwarks of support – in this case facilitated by the fact that the hospitals mostly took on charitable status for tax and legal purposes. At the same time, the entry of corporations and mutual societies into the health arena was checked, while the medical profession itself became an ever more influential player in shaping the organizational structure of the private hospital sector. Nor did federal, state or local government emerge strongly in this period as a countervailing power to offset the market position of physicians in terms of health insurance, given the stable, politically liberal and decentralized nature of American society. Against this backcloth, in the words of Starr (1982: 232), the medical profession at this time 'helped shape the medical system so that its structure supported professional sovereignty instead of undermining it'. As we shall see, this shaping of the medical system is well illustrated by the role that the emergent federal Food and Drugs Administration played in protecting the boundaries of the American medical profession against external encroachment from alternative practitioners and others (Burrow 1963).

For the moment, it is important to note that the changes that occurred did not generally move the United States system in the more egalitarian direction that the British National Health Service was beginning to take at this time, as is very apparent from the work of Starr (1982). He highlights the widening inequalities in the geographical distribution of physicians between states, and between urban and rural areas, in the early years of the twentieth century. He also notes the overcrowding of the smaller numbers of public and charitable hospitals as compared with the relative underutilization of the profusion of predominantly fee-based private hospitals that grew up in the first few decades of the century. This process tended to work to the disadvantage of the less well off, despite the fact that charitable places were available in private hospitals. Weiss (1997) suggests that the interests of physicians also obstructed the development of public health measures, as they created competition for fee-paying patients who might no longer come to their office practices. The inequalities in the system were clear too from the low proportion of members of minority groups in the medical profession in the United States at that time. The position of women in this regard reflected to some degree the situation in Britain (Stacey 1985). While the leaders of the American Medical Association can be castigated for doing little to address such inequalities (see, for instance, Krause 1996), the very existence of these inequalities was an indicator of the growing power of organized medicine in the health care marketplace.

This power is underlined by the use of political influence by the American Medical Association to block proposals for publicly funded health insurance in the first part of the twentieth century (Heirich 1998). However, as Starr (1982) notes, the sovereignty that was gained in a predominantly private system – with all its strengths and weaknesses from the viewpoint of the consumer – was increasingly challenged in the 1930s and 1940s by the spectre of third-party intervention. Private health plans extending beyond direct services to employees, with a clear desire to limit costs, expanded significantly in this period. Physicians were especially wary of group health insurance schemes such as Blue Cross, because they feared encroachment on their territory and loss of professional authority. It is not surprising, therefore, that the American Medical Association held that such plans should accept monopoly control of the medical market by physicians, as well as their authority over medical institutions – although this authority was not always respected in practice. Nevertheless, the proactive stance of the American Medical Association and the local medical societies limited the threat from private health plans, including those offered by commercial insurers (Maioni 1998). This was achieved by reaching an accommodation with providers, while still meeting the interests of the predominantly middle-class subscribers, who were challenged by the sharply rising costs of medical care (Anderson 1989).

As Starr (1982) observes, the threat that developed from the 1930s onwards was mainly a result of medicine's own success. Among other things, it was necessary to spread the cost of medical care, which was increasingly prized, to ensure that it was affordable. In the end, the market position of physicians in the first half of the twentieth century was strengthened by confidence in the development of 'scientific' biomedicine, based largely on the bacteriological revolution. This made a significant impact in the United States, as in Britain. The quest for agents to kill germs led to the widespread application of the 'magic bullet', including sulpha drugs and penicillin. Bacteriological developments also led public health officials to adopt a more focused approach to water- and food-borne diseases, and prompted the development of vaccines against typhoid and tetanus. The introduction of antisepsis brought down mortality rates and extended the range of surgery. Moreover, technological innovation led to a wider range of health instrumentation becoming available, including such devices as the electrocardiograph and the X-ray (see, among others, Brandt and Gardner 2000; Duffin 1999). According to Starr (1982), one consequence of such developments in medical science was that the public felt less able to deal with their own health problems – and became technically more dependent on physicians.

Whatever the merits of this view, the government was certainly more willing to put money into hospital construction, as it did, for example, through the Hill–Burton grant programme from the mid-1940s onwards in support of voluntary hospitals (Anderson 1989). The first half of the twentieth century in the United States was also a time of increasing privately endowed research in medical care (Berliner 1985a). Financial support was provided by private foundations such as the Rockefeller Institute for Medical Research and the universities, as well as by bodies such as the pharmaceutical companies. Later in this period, research gained more public support, not least through the seemingly ever-expanding federal funding of the National Institutes of Health. Under this impetus, the quality of clinical research in the United States came to outstrip that taking place in Europe (Dally 1997). The rising authority of physicians, associated with this high-quality research, seems to have been translated into greater legal privileges, income and social status – with high-prestige areas such as surgery becoming a popular career choice (Duffin 1999). A tone of optimism became established in this era, even if the more generic field of public health medicine continued to be professionally peripheral in the United States at this time (Weiss 1997), paralleling the position in Britain (Baggott 2000).

Such medical developments were also associated with the growth of specialization in the period up to the 1950s. This led to a majority of physicians having specialist roles, the proportion of whom came to far outstrip their counterparts in Britain as the century wore on (Stevens 1971). To grasp why this occurred, it is important to understand the different organizational structures in health care that developed in the United States. Patients were able to go directly to a specialist, as opposed to being permitted to consult a specialist only after being referred by a general practitioner, as in the British system (Fry 1969). Moreover, while the hospital as a site for treatment increased in importance in both countries, the United States did not adopt the rigid two-tier system that characterized British medicine, whereby general practitioners and specialists occupied distinct and largely impenetrable spheres. Instead, private medical practitioners in the community could gain access to hospitals without becoming employees – to such an extent that even by 1933, five out of every six physicians held hospital appointments. In this respect, unlike in Britain, hospital-based specialists in the United States failed to prevent general practitioners from engaging in specialty career development – even though the American Medical Association increasingly set minimum standards for hospital internships (Starr 1982).

It is interesting to note that by the 1920s, membership of local medical societies was the main informal prerequisite for joining the staff of most local hospitals, thereby increasing professional control over the hospital sector. Although by the 1930s a more systematic framework of certification by specialty boards had developed in relation to standards, such boards could not stop uncertified physicians from practising as specialists, or hospitals from giving admission privileges to non-certificated practitioners. Starr (1982) sees the consequent fluidity of the practice boundaries between the community and the hospital sector – coupled with the lack of a secure mediating role for the general practitioner – as the main factor in the increasing breakdown of traditional patterns of general practice in the United States. This fluidity, together with high market demand for specialist care, seems to have led to the massive growth of specialization in the United States. The upshot was the founding of many specialist examining boards, ranging from those for ophthalmology in 1916 and otolaryngology in 1924 to anaesthesiology in 1937 and thoracic surgery in 1948, with a total of nineteen boards having been formed by 1950 (Stevens 1971).

The even more substantial medical fragmentation to which this gave rise in the United States as compared to Britain did not necessarily weaken the power of the profession. The burgeoning specialization was overseen from the 1930s onwards not only by the American Medical Association Council on Medical Education, but also by the related Advisory Board for Medical Specialties (Stevens 1971). Starr (1982) also suggests that the need for mutual referrals between practitioners and hospital privileges in this system made physicians more corporate in outlook as they became more dependent on colleagues than on clients – enabling their collective rather than their individual interests to prevail. The development of medical training according to the values and standards of specialists further strengthened the American medical profession, moreover, in a system much influenced by biomedical research. In this respect, as Starr notes, the reconstitution of the hospital made it more central to medical education, as it was increasingly transformed from a place of impurity and exile to a 'citadel of science'. Hospitals provided a strong clinical framework for medical education as links with medical schools developed, the numbers of research-based staff of which had also expanded significantly by the mid-twentieth century. This expansion highlights the academic standing and power of the ever more specialized medical profession at this time.

THE EMERGENCE OF THE PROFESSIONS ALLIED TO MEDICINE IN THE UNITED STATES

As Krause (1996) observes, this power was also manifested in the licensing boards in medicine in individual states, which worked under the control of the state medical associations in carrying out the policies of the profession. The licensing boards were very significant in the relationship to other orthodox health professions that increasingly emerged. Krause points out that – as in Britain – the medical profession had consolidated its power over most of these health professions by the decades on either side of the mid-twentieth century. He notes that in so doing, it used its monopoly powers in particular states, in conjunction with the national Council on Medical Education, to accredit and sponsor compatible non-medical health programmes in the university sector.

Its tactics in this field in the case of areas such as nursing, X-ray technology, physical therapy and occupational therapy were to lobby state legislatures for approval of the relevant licensing laws, albeit with practice being allowed only under the supervision of a licensed physician. In some cases, the relationship of control that was established was reinforced by physician representation on the licensing boards of the group in question. The right of representation could be seen as a trade-off – in which the professionalization of allied health occupations was sponsored in exchange for acceptance of explicit medical domination. The allied occupations assumed a position of occupational 'subordination' in the health care division of labour in terms of the typology set out by Turner (1995), as in the British case.

According to Krause (1996), the other side of the coin based on medical interests was that national and state medical associations would not normally support the licensure of those health occupations that sought independence from the medical profession in the division of labour. These included their rivals in alternative medicine, whom – as we shall see in the next chapter – they typically actively and vigorously opposed. To have allowed them independence would have been to reduce the medical profession's control of the occupational structure in health care and open the field up to increased competition, with all the associated threats to medical income, status and power. Dentists, however, proved to be an exception to this rule in the United States, as in Britain. They were usually given an exclusive licence to practise in their restricted field, which provided for the prosecution of unlicensed competitors (Freidson 1986) – although there were demarcation disputes with physicians in the mid-twentieth century over such matters as who had responsibility for surgery of the jaw (Stevens 1971). Optometrists also found themselves in a comparable position as independent practitioners, following battles with the ophthalmologists in a relatively lucrative field of practice (Starr 1982). As in the British context, they were bound by the limits of their own expertise – creating a 'limited', rather than a fully fledged, profession within the terms outlined by Turner (1995).

Medical dominance of the health care division of labour in the United States was also accentuated in specific organizational contexts, particularly in relation to the subordinated professions allied to medicine. As Krause (1996) remarks, American hospitals in this period were usually under the doctors' control, with departments being effectively run by a chief who generally was a private practising physician. Although most auxiliary health professionals were employed by the hospital and could receive conflicting instructions from other hospital managers, they tended to work directly under the orders of a doctor. In office settings too they typically worked on a salary for physicians, who had the authority to define illness – and did not accept the right of other health occupations to do so (Freidson 1970). This set-up in large part mirrored the situation in Britain in the first half of the twentieth century, where doctors had independent control of allied health professionals in the division of labour as private contractors in general practice. Medical consultants also tended to call the shots in this respect in the hospitals in the private, voluntary and public sectors in this period, despite the far-reaching reforms that were occurring in the structure of national health provision at this time (Stacey 1988).

This medical dominance of an increasingly elaborate division of labour in the United States largely dated from the professionalization of medicine at the turn of the century. Starr (1982) notes that nurses had established in excess of one thousand nursing schools by 1910 in their quest for professionalization. The form of the state-based licensure that they increasingly achieved was heavily shaped by their turf battle with physicians (Kalisch and Kalisch 1995). This is highlighted by the fact that before the 1920s, nurses sometimes fulfilled the role of anaesthetists as there were too few physicians, a position that was no longer considered acceptable with the rise of anaesthesiology as a major specialty in medicine. It is noteworthy too from the viewpoint of the politics of professionalization that in the period up to the 1930s, nurses divided themselves into a pecking order of registered nurses, licensed practical nurses and nurses' aides (Freidson 1970). The hierarchical manner in which they did this mirrored the relationship that developed between physicians and nurses and other subordinated professions allied to medicine in this period. There is a parallel in the way in which British nurses progressively shed such 'dirty work' as emptying bedpans and cleaning the wards from the Nightingale era onwards as part of the process of professionalization (Garmarnikow 1978).

Such politicized processes in the search for ever greater professional standing relative to medicine in the first fifty years of the twentieth century are well illustrated by the growing specialization and the increasingly lengthy undergraduate programmes in nursing in the United States as the 1950s approached (Duffy 1979). This was one of a number of areas in which the relationship between non-physician and physician groups was highly sensitive. Another was the gender-based interface between obstetricians and midwives, in which – as in Britain – midwives were significantly disadvantaged through the restrictive role created by the regulatory legislation that was enacted (Donnison 1977). American midwives, however, typically had fewer technical skills than their European counterparts and had not developed a consolidated national base (Stevens 1971). In this context, their numbers went into sharp decline in the conflict with physicians as state after state legislated against them in favour of the obstetricians in the early years of the twentieth century (Ehrenreich and English 1973). Such legislation drove midwives almost to the point of extinction, as they increasingly assumed the mantle of alternative practitioners. They did survive, though, in some lower-income rural areas that were not well served by physicians (Stevens 1971), but no longer represented the same level of challenge posed by other occupational groups in the health care division of labour.

In cases where there was a more consistent challenge, other potentially competing groups within medical orthodoxy in the United States tended to be subordinated to the doctors' authority, or otherwise controlled through formal territorial restrictions in the division of labour. Two groups that became subordinated in this way were X-ray technicians and laboratory workers, who far outnumbered radiologists and pathologists, but whose function cut across these key medical specialisms. As Stevens (1971) indicates, the physicians concerned not only successfully sought specialist recognition in the 1930s, but also employed the tactic of ensuring that the development of hospital facilities for such groups took place under their control. Qualified technicians and technologists were registered as separate categories of personnel under their own professional umbrellas. To achieve professional qualification required them to follow a prescribed pattern of training and adhere to a code of ethics stipulating that they would work only under the supervision of a qualified physician. In consequence, physicians were generally able to ensure that X-ray technicians and laboratory workers did not practise independently, or give their interpretation of X-rays or tests directly to patients.

There are therefore many similarities with Britain as regards the expanding health care division of labour – even if it is important to acknowledge differences between these countries over such issues as the time-spans within which particular allied professional groups gained the right to licensing and registration (Larkin 2000). There are also debates parallel to those outlined in relation to Britain, about why the American medical profession managed to gain and maintain its position of dominance over other health occupations in the orthodox division of labour by the 1950s. The classic functionalist work of Parsons (1954) assumes the utility of modern scientific medicine in maintaining the capacity to perform social roles. This prerequisite for the functioning of the social system is held to account not only for the professionalization of medicine, but also for the physicians' place at the zenith of the American health care pecking order. However, there is a tension between this explanation and that of the neo-Weberians. Starr (1982: 144) captures this in relation to the consolidation of the position of members of the medical profession as follows:

The functionalist ascribes their advance to the growing importance of professional skills and technical knowledge, while the power theorist cites the monopolistic practices of the professions. In the case of medicine, the former sees the growth of valid medical knowledge as the key to the advance of the profession, while the latter finds an explanation in the profession's monopolization of that knowledge.

The conclusion reached by Starr (1982) in the face of this dichotomy is that the development of scientific knowledge was not sufficient in its own right to explain the position achieved by the medical profession in the United States by the mid-twentieth century. It is not sufficient because that position did not automatically transfer into authority and market power. At the same time, he notes that the impulse to achieve monopolistic power alone is not enough to explain the success or failure of any occupational group to articulate its own interests over competing interests. He therefore argues that the dominant market position of American medicine relates to lay deference and institutionalized forms of dependence, which sustain its authority. This argument, though, still risks reifying the role of 'scientific' progress in the success of medicine – which, as we shall see, poses empirical as well as philosophical problems in the light of the growing critique of orthodox biomedicine in recent years (Saks 1998a). It is also flawed, as Starr does not adequately recognize the importance of gender issues within a patriarchal society. In this regard, in 1940 more than 95 per cent of all American medical graduates were men – in contrast to the preponderantly female membership of most of the auxiliary health professions within medical orthodoxy at this time (Duffy 1979).

Navarro (1986) has also criticized Starr (1982) for placing too much emphasis, in explaining their dominance, on the power of physicians to persuade the wider American public of the value of their knowledge and skills. From a Marxist frame of reference, Navarro sees his analysis as legitimating the capitalist establishment and obscuring the repressive influence of the dominant capitalist class through the state, by ascribing too much to the will of the public. In this respect, it is certainly helpful explicitly to acknowledge the relevance of the capitalist context in charting the development of medical orthodoxy in the market conditions prevailing in the United States. Equally, it is important to note the significance of state power, which, as Berlant (1975) emphasizes, was fundamental to not only the initial professionalization of medicine, but also the conversion of monopolistic legal privileges into market advantages in the Anglo-American context. However, this acknowledgement does not sustain the self-fulfilling structural straitjacket of interpretation that Navarro advocates. As we saw in the British context earlier in this chapter, such an interpretation gives too little consideration to the influence of the interests of professional groups and the subtleties involved in charting the political role of the state.

This point is highlighted in relation to the United States by Krause (1996: 32), who observes:

> Professional associations, and the overall guild power of American medicine ..., grew from the 1930s to the early 1960s. Although World War II led to a closer working relationship between large corporations and the central state, it did not disturb in this time period, the essentially private model of American professions, nor their private power to control and accredit their training programs. Lobbying in Washington, professional associations repelled new federal threats to their autonomy.

Krause (1996: 32) interestingly goes on to argue that: 'Many new semi-professions established licensing between 1930 and 1960, but most never developed a fraction of the guild control of medicine ... to control all workplaces, expel competitors, and build a private market for services.' This relative lack of power testifies to the dominance of the medical profession in the health sector in the United States and the subjugated position of allied health professional groups in the period up to the mid-twentieth century. What, though, of the relationship between orthodox and alternative medicine in Britain and the United States in this period? The next chapter addresses this question more explicitly.

CHAPTER 3

The marginalization of alternative medicine

By the mid-twentieth century, the medical profession in both Britain and the United States had become a very strong force, as the empire of medical orthodoxy was consolidated and further elaborated with the rise of biomedicine. Although the form of the monopoly in part reflected the different societal contexts in which the profession was located, the consequences for health care practices that were henceforth defined as alternative medicine were similar on both sides of the Atlantic. They became viewed within the newly forged profession as what Wolpe (1994) conceptualizes as 'heresy': marginal beliefs that challenge the dominant orthodox ideology. In these terms, the leaders of the medical profession were involved in fighting the 'heretics' from within – and, even more importantly, the 'infidels' from without. In this encounter, as Wolpe makes plain, those marginalized were not just passive victims of orthodox strategies. They also developed strategies of their own, partly as a response to the actions of medical orthodoxy.

This process of marginalization marked the transcendence of the more pluralistic pre-industrial era leading up to the nineteenth century in the Anglo-American context, described in Chapter 1 of this book. These years can be characterized in terms of the ideal type set out by Cant and Sharma (1999) as involving a multiplicity of players competing on a more or less level playing field. As we saw in Chapter 2, this period was increasingly left behind following the professionalization of medicine, based on the 1858 Medical Registration Act in Britain and a flurry of state licensing laws passed around the turn of the century in the United States. Following this watershed, the antagonism towards competitors that had been evident in establishing the medical monopoly was perpetuated in the drive to maintain and extend the privileges of the profession. The consequent marginalization of alternative medicine, which will now be documented, was primarily based on 'exclusion' from the orthodox division of labour, as opposed to 'subordination' or 'limitation' within it, drawing on the categories set out by Turner (1995). This chapter, again written from a neo-Weberian perspective, focuses on the nature of the response of the medical profession to such therapies and the implications for patterns of alternative practice up to the 1950s.

Before we examine the trends in this period in more detail, it is worth reiterating that 'alternative medicine' is defined here in terms of its political marginality, as outlined in the Introduction. It is seen not so much in terms of its intrinsic characteristics, as of the relative lack of state support for its diverse forms in Britain and the United States. The diversity of alternative medicine means that it is sometimes helpful in the analysis to distinguish the specific therapies involved, as well as particular groups of practitioners subscribing to these. In considering the dynamics of the process, it should be emphasized that the medical profession itself is not always best viewed as a homogeneous entity. As was indicated in Chapter 2, medical orthodoxy in the Anglo-American context increasingly encompassed significant subdivisions in the period up to the mid-twentieth century, including that between general practitioners and specialists. Leaving aside the growing span of allied health professions, which were generally under fairly tight control in this period, it is also crucial to appreciate the importance of the hierarchical division between the élite and the rank and file in the medical profession (Saks 1995b). In addition, the perennial existence of 'heretics' in the ranks of orthodox medicine adds a further dimension to the account. Now that these analytical parameters have been set out, the position of alternative medicine in relation to medical orthodoxy can be considered in Britain and the United States in turn over the time-span concerned.

ALTERNATIVE MEDICINE IN BRITAIN UP TO THE MID-TWENTIETH CENTURY

THE MEDICAL RESPONSE TO ALTERNATIVE MEDICINE IN THE SECOND HALF OF THE NINETEENTH CENTURY

In Britain the state-legitimated professional boundaries that were established through the 1858 Medical Registration Act provided a sound basis for initially intensifying the attack on the various types of therapies being practised outside the profession. These were now officially categorized as unorthodox medicine – which gave firmer meaning to the concept of 'quackery' applied to rival practices in the more pluralistic structure that had existed prior to the mid-nineteenth century (Porter 2001). As we have seen, aside from the creation of a formally unified medical profession, the powers of medicine in the new order were strengthened by the introduction of exclusive, legal rights to the title of doctor, self-regulation, suing for fees, and state employment (Waddington 1984). This gave the medical establishment the formal tools to enhance its position further. From a neo-Weberian viewpoint, the interest of the profession as a whole now lay in defending and extending the income, status and power that it had won in the process of professionalization, particularly against 'quack' outsiders. Its attempts to do so led to a significant struggle between orthodox and unorthodox medicine in the period up to the turn of the century – at a stage when its professional privileges could still have been withdrawn in face of the continued existence of the 'levelling forces of liberalism and egalitarianism' (Berlant 1975: 167).

The threat from practitioners of alternative medicine

The greatest threat to the position of the medical profession at this time came from non-medical exponents of alternative medicine. They were still permitted to practise under the common law. Moreover, they had every incentive to do so, given the buoyant market that continued to exist for a number of years for the more popular alternative therapies in the private sector. The threat was sharpened for the profession by the fact that richer clients – including members of the nobility and royalty – had much interest in using alternative medicine, especially as it was often seen as a gentler alternative to the heroic therapies that were still prevalent in orthodox medicine (Nicholls 1988). Such markets also provided a financial temptation to members of the profession themselves to enter this field, particularly since the blurred divisions between 'regular' and 'irregular' practices that had existed in the first half of the nineteenth century continued into the period immediately beyond the mid-nineteenth century (Porter 2001). Doctors who employed alternative therapies heightened the threat to orthodox medical interests, both in their own right as competitors and still more so through the potential legitimation they gave to external rivals to the profession.

The threat from outsiders to collective medical interests arose partly from the challenge posed to the status and power of the profession by two main groups of practitioners making wide-ranging therapeutic claims, whose very existence endangered the exclusive knowledge base of the profession. The first group consisted of non-medically qualified 'empirics', whose practice was not rooted either in formal training or in a systematic body of theoretical knowledge. The second group comprised those subscribing to conflicting theories of health care, including such practitioners as the homoeopaths and naturopaths (Saks 1996). These groups threatened the 'scientific' knowledge that was in the process of being consolidated through medical education.

However, the challenge from alternative practitioners outside orthodox ranks in the second part of the nineteenth century was strongly accentuated by the potential fee loss to doctors in an overcrowded profession. To understand the extent of this threat, it needs to be recalled that low income remained endemic in the medical profession in many areas of the country – and especially among general practitioners, who were most vulnerable to competition (Porter 1995).

This financial aspect helps to explain why the profession did not generally approve of the lenient treatment of alternative therapists (Jones 1981). Such 'heretics' and 'infidels', though, frequently strove to defend their position in the market against orthodox medicine in this period. Herbalists, for instance, made claims about the superior safety and efficacy of their remedies (Brown 1985). Colleague-based publication and other networks helped to sustain such outlying belief systems among groups of alternative practitioners. Nicholls (1988) observes that in homoeopathy alone in the 1860s there were two quarterly journals and three monthly publications, not to mention a regularly updated directory of homoeopathic practitioners. In attacking the medical profession through these and other mechanisms, however, unorthodox practitioners invited further disparaging attention from orthodox medicine. This was particularly so in the sensitive decades following the mid-nineteenth century when the newly established professional monopoly was at its most fragile, not least because of the difficulties that had been experienced in gaining approval for the underpinning legislation through the parliamentary process (Waddington 1984).

Defending orthodox medical interests: the empire strikes back

In line with the broadly defined self-interests of its members, the leaders of the medical profession responded to these threats by endeavouring to suppress deviant insiders and by waging an ongoing campaign against outsiders associated with alternative medicine (Saks 1996). Central to the control that the medical profession sought to achieve at this time was the developing medical élite comprising leading figures in the British Medical Association and the Royal Colleges. Despite simmering internal conflicts between these bodies, they managed to adopt a number of effective strategies against alternative therapists. These ranged from engaging in negative invective about such practitioners outside the profession, to maintaining a close check on those entering its ranks and striking deviant insiders off the register (Saks 1995b). In carrying these strategies through, they were able to draw on increasing colleague solidarity, as the then fledgling profession developed in the period up to the turn of the century and beyond. This solidarity derived in large part from the exclusionary closure on which the profession was based. It was particularly fostered by the unifying arrangements that were introduced through the General Medical Council in relation to such areas as registration and the undergraduate medical curriculum, based on the orthodox biomedical paradigm (Stacey 1988).

Such growing professional unity – coupled with the decline of influence of the patronage system that had so shaped earlier health care practices (Jewson 1974) – also increased the social distance between medicine and competing bodies of health knowledge in this period. This distance was reinforced by the continuing development of professional journals such as the *British Medical Journal* that acted as major vehicles for debate and defined the normative boundaries of the medical community (Bartrip 1990). The definition of this community became tighter as the century wore on, with growing centralized control in élite hands and the ever-strengthening ideological link between the medical profession and the prestigious mantle of science (Saks 1995b). Moreover, while the fast-expanding proprietary medical sector largely associated itself with medical orthodoxy for commercial reasons (Vaughan 1959), much alternative practice in this period was based on the more personal, individualized approaches to treatment so much in vogue in earlier times. This further sharpened the differentiation from orthodox medicine, as illustrated by the cases of herbalism and homoeopathy in Victorian Britain (Brown 1987; Nicholls 1988).

The legitimacy that the profession increasingly drew from state support on the basis of its *de facto* monopoly (Berlant 1975) also helped orthodox medicine to demarcate its boundaries – to the detriment of alternative practice. The control of alternative therapies was further facilitated by the decision of the General Medical Council to limit the cooperation of doctors with unorthodox outsiders through its formal ethical codes, which checked its development (Inglis 1980). Unqualified practitioners were subjected to a barrage of criticism too from medical journals such as the *Lancet* in the latter half of the nineteenth century. This journal, for example, commented on 'the crass stupidity' of sick persons who 'place themselves in the hands of men who rob their victims of both money and life' (Lancet 1871: 598). It also distinguished the scientific 'rationality' of the medically qualified from the scientific 'irrationality' of alternative therapists (Lancet 1889). Such attacks enabled doctors to position themselves as representatives of a profession safeguarding the health needs of the wider public, in contrast to their unorthodox competitors, who were tainted with the charge of engaging in superstitious practices in an increasingly secular society (Saks 1999a).

The attack made by the British medical journals on non-medically qualified practitioners in the nineteenth century was extended to members of the public involved in fringe self-help activities. This covered many of the users of the range of preparations produced by the patent medicine industry, from pills and potions to balms and elixirs (Bartrip 1990). The attack also focused on treatments such as hydrotherapy, including water-based remedies at spas. Hydrotherapy, however, seems to have been regarded as less pernicious by the medical profession than other alternative practices such as vegetarianism, phrenology and mesmerism – perhaps because of the more extensive involvement of physicians in these areas and their greater incompatibility with heroic forms of orthodox medicine (Rees 1988). There was also negative medical reaction to the challenging popular practice of Baunscheidtism, which had spread to many parts of Europe by the mid-nineteenth century as a cure for all ills. This was based on the employment of a device with spring-attached needles that were used to create eruptions on the skin, centred on the traditional systems theory of disease. The sceptical posture of the profession was consistent with its shifting response at this time to other rudimentary forms of acupuncture being used by the medically unqualified to gain business from those suffering from such sexual complaints as impotence and irritation of the urethra (Lu Gwei-Djen and Needham 1980).

The medical élite attacked deviant medical practitioners too, whose ignorance and non-scientific orientation was felt to lower 'the dignity' of the profession, at a time when it was seeking to distinguish itself from competitors. Such overt criticism was a strong deterrent to the involvement of doctors in unorthodox health care, given its potentially negative implications for career progression, as medicine became more hospital based and 'scientifically' oriented (Saks 1995b). Informal colleague group controls such as ostracism were frequently employed in order to limit medical involvement in more threatening types of alternative medicine. Nicholls (1988) notes that medical practitioners of homoeopathy were often reluctant to reveal their identity as sanctions of this kind began to bite, in spite of the existence of homoeopathic hospitals and dispensaries. Such was the strength of feeling against the insider practice of homoeopathy that some doctors who practised it lost their hospital posts, and one doctor was refused a Fellowship of the Edinburgh College of Physicians. The tactics of the medical élite generally were to attack the character of homoeopaths, publicize instances where homoeopathy had failed to produce results, and provide theoretical critiques of this system of therapy.

There is also evidence that in the second half of the nineteenth century the medical establishment was instrumental in blocking attempts by more organized groups of alternative practitioners to gain the legitimacy provided by formal recognition from the state. Griggs (1997), for instance, notes that the National Association of Medical Herbalists – which has now become the

National Institute of Medical Herbalists – battled for a charter in the 1890s that would have given its members the standing of registered practitioners. However, it was turned down as a result of bitter opposition from the medical profession, leaving the Association to settle for registration as a limited company. According to Griggs (1997: 234), the Association's failure to gain a charter marked a further stage in the history of herbalism of the 'continuous record of harassment, vexation and attempted legal suppression by the medical establishment'. As a result, its members remained legally debarred under the 1858 Medical Registration Act from such activities as giving medical evidence in the courts, holding medical appointments, providing sickness notes or signing death certificates – even though herbalists apparently commanded considerable public support at this time.

ALTERNATIVE THERAPIES IN RETREAT IN THE FIRST HALF OF THE TWENTIETH CENTURY

The above example highlights the effects of the medical onslaught on the interests of alternative practitioners in terms of income, status and power by the start of the twentieth century in Britain. The numbers of such therapists appear to have declined quite considerably at this time, as indicated by the *Report as to the Practice of Medicine and Surgery by Unqualified Persons in the United Kingdom* (1910). This trend, moreover, seems to have continued – and perhaps accelerated – in the first half of the twentieth century. In this period, the fragmented cluster of alternative practitioners outside the medical profession became further disadvantaged by the passing of the 1911 National Health Insurance Act and the 1946 National Health Service Act, which reinforced the *de facto* monopoly of the profession (Berlant 1975). As we have seen, these reforms placed the medical profession in an even more pre-eminent position as a supplier of health services in the greatly expanded state sector. This position was underlined by the exclusivity that doctors had obtained through the 1858 Act over appointments to public office (Porter 1995), which meant that non-medically qualified alternative practitioners were confined to the increasingly marginalized private market.

As was noted in Chapter 2, the inequalities in public access to such therapies that resulted need to be viewed against the rising legitimacy of modern medicine, gained primarily through its still growing scientific reputation. The further expansion of the unity of the profession with educational reform and increasing state support enhanced its power, as the evolving split into general practitioners and specialists was bridged with the development of the referral system. This also meant that it was even easier to differentiate the medical profession and the increasing numbers of allied health occupations from outsiders (Stevens 1966). These changes further advanced medical interests in relation to alternative medicine in the first half of the twentieth century, as the monopolistic position of the profession became more and more secure. While they did not totally drive alternative practice out of existence in Britain in this period, it had largely faded from view by the 1950s. Both non-medical and medical practitioners of such therapies, as well as their self-help use, became virtually invisible in the public and private sectors – with all the implications that this carried for consumer access to alternative medicine (Saks 1995b).

The struggle of the medical profession against 'quack' remedies

Skirmishes nonetheless continued between orthodox and unorthodox medicine throughout the first half of the twentieth century in Britain. These were nowhere more apparent than in the struggle of the profession at this time against 'quack' remedies, from cures for gout and consumption, to revitalizing tonic wines and pills to produce abortions. The use of such remedies among the public had grown from their more restricted application in the nineteenth century to high levels of employment in the early years of the twentieth century. The battle here began in the late 1880s, but had substantially intensified by the turn of the century. Vaughan (1959) notes that this struggle was manifested in the campaign that the British Medical Association waged to have the contents of all patent medicines printed on the labels they carried. As part of this campaign, the British Medical Journal regularly published its own exposures of the composition of different forms of secret remedies. These were eventually collected together into two volumes on this subject (British Medical Association 1909, 1912). Here it was claimed that the vast majority of secret remedies were worthless and many were actively dangerous because of their ingredients – while, in addition, their use might lead to crucial delays in seeking medical advice.

Vaughan (1959) stresses that this action could be seen as in the interests of the medical profession, in the light of the multi-million-pound trade in 'quack' medicines at this time – sustained by the newspaper industry, which benefited greatly from the ensuing advertising revenues. The extent of the challenge to the income, status and power of the medical profession was accentuated by the fact that the remedies covered conditions of all conceivable kinds. Unorthodox practitioners too were often involved in both providing diagnoses and prescribing treatments associated with such remedies, usually on a postal basis. In addition, the remedies themselves were given a spurious official legitimation by the stamp that had to be placed on the packaging to confirm that stamp duty was being paid to the government. Although public health benefits were doubtless gained from the campaign by the British Medical Association against some of the more outlandish types of secret remedies, sight should not be lost of the professional self-interests involved, in a highly competitive environment (Saks 1995b). These also included those of pharmacists, who supported the medical profession in its actions against its rivals in the patent medicine business by taking legal action where necessary (Bartrip 1990).

The recommendations of the Select Committee that was set up in 1912 to investigate patent medicines and foods, partly as a result of the campaign by the British Medical Association, are interesting in this light. While accepting in its 1914 report that further measures were needed to regulate the sector, it stopped short of recommending that the composition of 'quack' remedies be publicly displayed because they were trade secrets (Vaughan 1959). Nonetheless, the Association's campaign prompted a range of subsequent legislation that further reined in fringe competitors, as the link between profession and state grew closer (Larkin 1995). This legislation included the 1917 Venereal Disease Act, which banned the advertisement and sale of remedies in this field, as well as restrictions introduced in the 1920s on the use of substances such as opium and cocaine in such medicines. Additional legislation in the 1930s and 1940s, as a result of lobbying by the leaders of the medical profession, limited the claims that could be made in other areas. In this respect, the 1939 Cancer Act stopped non-registered medical practitioners from treating or offering to treat cancer, while the 1941 Pharmacy and Medicines Act placed similar controls over conditions such as cataracts, diabetes, glaucoma, epilepsy and tuberculosis (Vaughan 1959).

The medical response to the diminishing challenge from alternative practitioners

By its very nature, this legislation struck further at non-medical practitioners of alternative medicine. Certain groups of alternative therapists, moreover, continued to be specifically attacked in the medical journals. A good example is the case of the osteopaths, who were subjected to derision for having 'far-fetched and fanciful' theories that were 'decidedly dangerous' when applied to serious diseases (Larkin 1992). The extent to which particular groups of alternative therapists were subjected to attack seems to have been largely linked to the degree of threat they posed to the interests of the medical profession. The view of many osteopaths that most disorders were explicable in terms of spinal irregularities, which could be corrected by manipulation, put them into competition with medicine on a broad front. This was accentuated by the fact that they were a very active group. The assault on unorthodox outsiders, though, was generally far less proactively pursued in the mainstream medical journals in the first half of the twentieth century than previously, as the challenge from such practitioners diminished in the face of growing professional dominance (Saks 1995b).

This growing dominance is illustrated by the sharp downturn in the numbers of items on acupuncture in the *British Medical Journal* and the *Lancet* from the turn of the century onwards, following a steady decrease in the latter half of the nineteenth century. The fact that this subject was barely mentioned in these journals at this time correlates with the diminishing challenge that non-medical acupuncturists presented to the income, status and power of the medical profession, as their numbers and presence declined (Saks 1991b). While favourable reports about acupuncture may have been screened out by the journals concerned, it does not seem to have been considered worthwhile any more to scapegoat practitioners in this field (Saks 1995b). The medical attack on mesmerism also subsided as it became superseded by the turn of the century by the more professionally respectable practice of hypnotism, which was generally confined to medical practitioners. Hypnotism was not the threatening popular culture phenomenon that mesmerism had been for much of the nineteenth century, when it was seen as resembling healing by touch, which was felt to be based on ancient superstitions. Thus, it no longer significantly challenged the scientific respectability of the medical profession, its theoretical rationale or the income of its practitioners (Parssinen 1979).

Herbalists, however, showed that the threat to the medical profession from non-medical practitioners of alternative medicine had not totally disappeared by the first half of the twentieth century. The National Association of Medical Herbalists put forward two bills in the 1920s proposing a Herbalists' Council to train and register its members, without medical oversight (Larkin 1995). The Association also advocated that herbalists should receive payment for treating patients under the National Health Insurance Act – their exclusion from which had surprised its practitioners, especially as after 1911 growing numbers of local insurance companies had refused to offer contracts to them (Griggs 1997). This attempt to gain state sanction for their activities, paralleling that of doctors, highlights the degree of competitive challenge that they posed to medical interests. The challenge was amplified by their belief in the broad therapeutic applicability of herbalism. However, as Larkin (1995) notes, the medical profession was able to bring about the rejection of the proposals from the herbalists as the General Medical Council was given a central role by the government in offering it medical advice, based on its growing authority.

The threat from herbalists should not be exaggerated, though, as the National Association of Medical Herbalists could not even at this stage sustain a school of herbalism for training its members – instead mainly relying on postal courses. Against this, there was considerable support among politicians for its cause (Griggs 1997). Similar support was offered when the British and Incorporated Associations of Osteopaths sought independent state registration with self-regulatory powers in the 1930s. Osteopathy was more challenging than herbalism at this stage because of the progress it had already made in gaining recognition in the United States and the greater cohesiveness of its practitioners as a group (Larkin 1995). The medical élite, however, had developed its role still further as the main arbiter of the boundaries of orthodox medicine. Operating as the key adviser to government, it was again able effectively to block the bills that were put forward. As in the case of the herbalists, therefore, the submissions that the osteopaths made were effectively thwarted by the medical–Ministry alliance.

The cases of the osteopaths and the herbalists highlight the fate of two groups that did not seek to advance their position under the umbrella of medical patronage, as neither wished to trade off subordination to medicine for state recognition (Larkin 1992; Griggs 1997). The result was that they remained marginal practitioners for the rest of the first half of the twentieth century and beyond. The threat of external encroachment on the monopoly rights of the profession was thereby averted in line with medical interests, largely because of its close links with the state. As we saw in Chapter 2, such links were also used to good effect in ensuring the supremacy of medicine in the face of the development of a range of professions allied to medicine at this time – from midwifery and nursing to physiotherapy and occupational therapy. In this case, however, the claim that scientific medicine was at odds with the dogmatic approach of the osteopaths and the herbalists served to exclude such practitioners from, rather than incorporate them into, orthodox medicine (Larkin 1995).

The medical establishment also used the powers that had been bestowed on it under the 1858 Medical Registration Act to control deviant practitioners within the profession, in order to protect its interests after the turn of the century. In this respect, those at the apex of the profession and those at the grassroots had the least to lose by taking up alternative practice, from a career viewpoint (Saks 1995b). As Inglis (1980) documents, the leverage that the medical élite was able to exercise over careers in the profession was particularly important. This leverage even seems to have held back Sir Thomas Horder from further researching the famous 'black box' of Albert Abrams, a widely ridiculed fringe device for making diagnoses from body samples. Despite the ridicule, the official inquiry that Horder had conducted in

1924 yielded positive results. Yet if the pursuit of his interest may have prevented Horder from becoming a peer, and physician to the king, doctors cooperating with alternative therapists at the other end of the scale in this period were struck off the medical register. The victims included the anaesthetist to Herbert Barker, the famous bonesetter. The controls exercised by the medical élite were also administered through gatekeepers policing such areas as entry to medical education, the acceptance of journal publications, and access to the growing levels of official research funding (Saks 1996).

These mechanisms – aided by the increasing power and unity of the medical profession – helped to keep alternative medicine in all its forms at the margins of health care in the first half of the twentieth century. In this regard, the prejudicial effects on the interests of alternative practitioners inside and outside the profession should be emphasized. Aside from their structural disadvantaged positions in relation to medical orthodoxy, such practitioners were typically stigmatized (Inglis 1980). Non-medically qualified alternative therapists were also usually relatively poorly rewarded as a result of their marginal status. The detrimental effects of the development of state medicine on their livelihoods were thrown into focus by protests in 1945 from the newly formed British Health and Freedom Society, which represented practices such as naturopathy and osteopathy, as well as herbalism (Larkin 1995). Similar difficulties also applied to those associated with alternative practice within the medical profession, who sometimes risked their jobs at a time when growing security was available in more orthodox, state-supported market shelters. The difficulties were exacerbated by the divisions between practitioners in this field, particularly among the non-medically qualified (Griggs 1997).

In the first half of the twentieth century, therefore, the interests of orthodox medicine prevailed over those of unorthodoxy in the politics of health care. A case in point is homoeopathy. Having been such a strong force in the latter half of the nineteenth century, this therapy, according to Nicholls (1988: 207), went into 'dramatic decline after the turn of the century'. This was reflected in the fact that by 1930, the cluster of homoeopathic practitioners in Britain had reduced to less than two hundred, as compared to close to forty thousand doctors. In addition, there was a steep decline in the numbers of homoeopathic hospitals and dispensaries up to the mid-twentieth century. This can be attributed to various factors, including opposition from the medical profession, as well as internal dissension. Much the same trends were evident in many other unorthodox fields, bringing alternative medicine to the brink of extinction in Britain (Saks 1995b).

This is not to say, though, that no progress was made at this time through the strategies adopted by exponents of the medical alternatives. Taking homoeopathy as an example again, medical homoeopaths were able to found the Faculty of Homoeopathy, which was recognized by the Board of Trade in 1943 (Nicholls 1988). This had the right, among other things, to set the standard for postgraduate educational programmes and examinations. Following political lobbying, royal assent was also obtained for the Faculty of Homoeopathy Act in 1950, which underwrote its postgraduate licensing powers. However, this achievement was not achieved without a struggle. The British Postgraduate Medical Federation had not been happy at first to approve the London Homoeopathic Hospital as a teaching hospital. Subsequently, deans of postgraduate medical education were not willing to fund postgraduate study in this area in the Faculty, which meant that students had to find their own funding or apply for assistance outside the public purse. Even this success story, therefore, had serious limits. It was also the exception that proved the rule. By the mid-twentieth century most alternative medicine had seriously declined and its practitioners were in retreat – in the face of the growing powers of the orthodox medical profession. How did this compare with the position of unorthodox therapies in the United States, following the professionalization of medicine at the beginning of the century?

ALTERNATIVE MEDICINE IN THE UNITED STATES UP TO THE MID-TWENTIETH CENTURY

THE MEDICAL RECEPTION OF ALTERNATIVE MEDICINE IN THE FIRST HALF OF THE TWENTIETH CENTURY

As in Britain, the boundaries of medical orthodoxy put in place both nationally and at state level in the United States served as a platform for attacking the practice of alternative medicine operating outside such parameters. Although the professionalization of medicine occurred at a later stage than Britain – from the turn of the century onwards – the American medical profession too was increasingly able to use the patchwork of licensure that was developed to advance its standing. In neo-Weberian terms, the medical establishment had interests in maintaining the legal exclusivity of the profession in the face of competitors in order to sustain and, wherever possible, expand its income, status and power. These interests may help to explain why, as was noted in Chapter 2, national and state medical associations did not typically support the independent licensure of health occupations outside medical orthodoxy. While groups such as nurses and other professions allied to medicine were kept within the fold, the leaders of the ever more unified medical profession were in conflict with non-medical practitioners of alternative medicine throughout the first half of the twentieth century.

The growing challenge from alternative practitioners

Unlike in Britain, where common law rights prevailed, in the United States it was technically illegal for medically unlicensed competitors to practise without there being a separate licensing board (Freidson 1986). This situation mitigated but did not remove the challenge posed by non-medical practitioners, not least because alternative therapists could establish their own licensing bodies with state sanction. These bodies did not exist for such unorthodox groups as acupuncturists, faith healers and naturopaths in the United States at the beginning of the century (Cohen 1998). However, they increasingly emerged as the twentieth century wore on (Saks 2000b), as epitomized by the osteopaths, who obtained licensing laws in the vast majority of states by the 1950s, despite medical opposition. Their success was in part orchestrated by the American Osteopathic Association, which had the explicit purpose from the time of its foundation in 1897 of securing professional recognition, with independent boards of registration and examination in every state. It even established at an early stage a permanent Committee on Legislation, as well as extending the length of undergraduate qualifications and promoting a code of ethics in order to achieve this end. The main aim was to gain greater autonomy and security in the face of orthodox medicine, in a period when the range of osteopathic training schools was expanding. Although not all the increasing numbers of osteopathic practitioners were members of the Association, the collective threat that osteopaths posed was significant (Gevitz 1982).

Another, even more challenging group of alternative practitioners for the American medical profession was the chiropractors, who were extremely committed to their cause, and were founded, like osteopathy, in the late nineteenth century. The numbers of these competing practitioners also grew rapidly in the early twentieth century, alongside the expansion of chiropractic colleges. As Wardwell (1988) relates, the first national organization in this area, the Universal Chiropractors' Association, was formed in 1906. This body was established largely to provide legal assistance to those practising chiropractic without a licence, in the face of medical persecution. It later split into the American Chiropractic Association and the International Chiropractors' Association, both of which sought to advance the standing of chiropractic – albeit with differing interpretations of the level of 'purity' with which this therapy should be delivered. As a result of lobbying, most states had passed legislation allowing chiropractors to be issued with licences by the middle of the twentieth century. Testimony to the challenge that they posed to orthodox medicine is that they often practised openly and extensively in states where they had not gained licensure, even though doing so potentially exposed them to legal sanction (Starr 1982).

Against this, as we have seen, even where they did win the right to practise, such alternative practitioners did not necessarily gain hospital access or drug prescribing rights in the first half of the twentieth century in the United States. Their numbers, moreover, were still relatively modest – comprising some thirty-six thousand practitioners who took care of little more than 5 per cent of all attended cases of illness by the end of the 1920s. They amounted to just over one-fifth of all physicians practising at this time (Starr 1982). This proportion was still threatening to the profession, especially in the case of some forms of alternative therapy with an affluent clientele, as their patronage of alternative practitioners increased financial competition for physicians from those both inside and outside the medical profession in a predominantly fee-for-service system. Such financial competition certainly applied to homoeopathy, for which there was a substantial demand from rich clients (Rothstein 1973), as in Britain. It was less true of chiropractic, where the emphasis on an active approach to illness was more in tune with working-class lifestyles, and particularly popular in rural settings that were less heavily populated by physicians (Wardwell 1992). Nonetheless, even here the threat to medical interests should not be underestimated, as medical earnings were not uniformly high, particularly for generalists (Stevens 1971). In addition, chiropractic challenged the profession of medicine, as it shared with homoeopathy a whole-system philosophy that contradicted the emerging biomedical orthodoxy (Gevitz 1988b).

The pursuit of medical interests against alternative practitioners

It is easy to understand, therefore, why the temporary unification with the homoeopaths and the eclectics around the turn of the century that facilitated the professionalization of American medicine described in Chapter 1 was swiftly brought to a conclusion. As previously noted, it was in the self-interests of physicians to forge an alliance with groups such as the homoeopaths against other competitors in this period, given the absence of a robust licensing system and strong public anti-trust sentiments. However, as Kaufman (1988) describes, once professionalization had been achieved, the leaders of the profession were able to outflank their erstwhile allies. After a number of abortive attempts between 1908 and 1913 by the American Medical Association and the American Institute of Homoeopathy to establish an 'unbiased' investigation of homoeopathy, it was seriously damaged by the Flexner medical reforms, which laid down minimum standards for the state licensing of medical schools. As we saw in Chapter 2, these reforms led the medical profession to close and/or reform many training establishments – including almost all the schools of homoeopathy. By 1922 only two such schools were in existence, and in 1935 the Council on Medical Education of the American Medical Association refused to include any institutions of 'sectarian medicine' on its list of approved schools and hospitals. This refusal signalled the decline of homoeopathy as a significant part of orthodox medicine – which was confirmed by the subsequent failure to recruit sufficient doctors to postgraduate homoeopathy courses.

Refusal to approve non-orthodox schools and hospitals was one of a number of measures that the American medical establishment was able to take up to the mid-twentieth century to defend its interests against unorthodox practitioners. In this respect, the threat that the profession was striving to counter largely came from the non-medically qualified (Gevitz 1988b). For example, one of the main challenges in this period emanated from the American Foundation for Homoeopathy, founded in 1921, which had a primarily lay membership (Kaufman 1988). As Starr (1982: 198) notes, at this stage 'medicine was still a beleaguered profession' in relation to 'unscientific sectarians and quacks'. As in Britain, the lay practitioners of alternative medicine with whom they were in competition could be divided into two major groups – the 'empirics', whose work was based on experience, and those with more training who subscribed to conflicting theories of medicine. For different reasons both provided a root-and-branch challenge to the income, status and power of the American medical profession, with its biomedical underpinnings in education and research. In this light, it is not surprising in terms of professional self-interests that the American Medical Association should have taken further aggressive steps to control outsiders (Burrow 1963).

These included the passing of legislation parallel to that of Britain to restrict exponents of 'quackery', for which individual states imposed limits on the practice of non-medically qualified unorthodox practitioners (Gevitz 1988b). As was noted earlier in this book, action was taken against female midwives, who gained a form of subordinated professional closure in Britain, but in the United States were outlawed by state after state, following attacks on them by obstetricians for being 'unscientific' and 'incompetent' (Ehrenreich and English 1973). The success of the obstetricians was based on the legally underwritten monopolistic strengths that the medical profession had gained in the marketplace. Wardwell (1994a: 1062) observes more generally that, to ensure that non-medical practitioners of alternative medicine were suitably constrained, the profession historically relied 'on the legislatures, the courts, and the police as the formal instruments of social control'. This control was complemented by 'informal procedures of excluding undesirables from membership in medical societies and hospital staffs'. In such ways, organized medicine did everything from prosecuting alternative practitioners for violating legislation concerning medical practice to denying alternative practitioners consultation rights and discouraging their patients from using such therapists (Gevitz 1988b). Thus the medical profession used a variety of strategies to control unorthodox outsiders, as in Britain.

In the first half of the twentieth century in the United States, however, the medical profession had more formal legal powers than in Britain to enforce its exclusivity in accord with its collective interests. These powers were employed against osteopathy, which also initially took a more challenging holistic approach to diagnosis and treatment (Ellis 1997). There was intense opposition from organized medicine to state support for its practice, which led to the exclusion of osteopaths from membership of, and cooperative relationships with, the medical profession. At a local level, the likelihood of prosecution depended in part on the extent to which osteopaths publicly proclaimed their superior skill as compared to those practising biomedicine. Where such practitioners presented an overtly competitive profile, they were more likely to be jailed for practising without a licence (Gevitz 1982). Chiropractors were also heavily targeted by medical orthodoxy. Many were arrested and imprisoned for the unlicensed practice of medicine. By 1927 the Universal Chiropractors' Association had dealt with some 3300 cases in the courts, with those put in jail assuming the status of martyrs for the chiropractic cause (Wardwell 1988). Prosecutions also occurred in a number of other areas of alternative medicine, albeit on a lesser scale, such as in Christian Science in states where its practitioners were not exempted from legislation related to medical licensing (Schoepflin 1988).

Much as in Britain, practitioners of unorthodox therapies were generally subjected to disparaging verbal assaults by leading figures in orthodox medicine. The labels of 'cultism' and 'quackery' were widely used by the American Medical Association to describe their activities. These were applied to a broad span of alternative therapy in the first half of the twentieth century, from Hamilton's drugless treatment of obesity based on diet and exercise to Hoxsey's cancer sanitarium, the proponents of which were seen as 'swindlers' by the medical establishment (Burrow 1963). As Gevitz (1988b) notes, for most doctors alternative therapists tended to fall into two categories: those who were 'deluded' or 'deranged' on the one hand and those who were 'charlatans' or 'imposters' on the other. In addition, supporters of medical orthodoxy highlighted the harm that could be caused by alternative medicine, from the negative effects of the toxic vitamins of the naturopaths and the cold baths of the hydropaths, to the deleterious consequences of the vigorous manipulation of osteopaths and chiropractors. Cases of disability and death directly arising from alternative medicine were widely reported in medical journals of the day. It was also argued that such therapies could indirectly cause harm by deterring patients from seeking more effective orthodox medical treatment (Wardwell 1988).

The desire of medical orthodoxy, however, seems to have generally been the same as in Britain – namely, to drive the 'infidels' out of practice. As a result, other groups associated with alternative medicine also faced the wrath of leaders of the American Medical Association, including members of the public who used such therapies – who were frequently attacked for their gullibility. Ministers of the Church too were even sometimes specifically castigated for using their influence to support 'medical fakes' and 'charlatans' (Burrow 1963). Gevitz (1988b: 14) observes that some physicians thought that 'given the scanty credentials of these quacks, their outrageous theories and doctrines, and their fantastic and unbelievable claims to cure, only the ignorant and simple-minded fell victim to their appeals'. However, he adds that since their clients included well-educated people of standing in the community, other members of the medical profession felt that such patients were 'simply not competent in medical matters' and did not have 'the necessary knowledge or background to be able to distinguish science from non-science'. In view of these perceptions, the medical establishment launched a major public education campaign to correct any misapprehensions, as part of its efforts to control the unorthodox.

Individual physicians who were tempted for financial and other reasons to use alternative medicine were also open to attack as 'heretics' within the profession, paralleling the case of Britain. In the first half of the twentieth century such physicians were able to practise alternative therapies in most states as long as they held a medical licence. However, issues of insurance eligibility, prescriptive ethical codes and the differential availability of research funding restricted their engagement with unorthodox therapies (Gevitz 1988b). Even research foundations that sponsored orthodox medicine where the patron was sympathetic to alternative therapies – such as the Rockefeller Foundation – did not lend support to this field (Berliner 1985a). These mechanisms were reinforced by ostracism by peers, including exclusion from local medical societies. In addition, those involved in unorthodox practice were disparagingly depicted in the columns of the medical journals (Gevitz 1988b). The *Journal of the American Medical Association*, for example, referred to such medical heretics as money-grabbing 'testio-maniacs', who illegitimately based their practice on spurious testimonials from clients (Burrow 1963). Such strategies were generally effective, given their potential impact on the future careers of physicians – particularly at a time when the profession more fully subscribed to the biomedical paradigm and its members were becoming more dependent on colleague referral networks as medical specialties developed (Freidson 1970).

One of the most prominent American physicians involved in this field in the early part of the twentieth century was Albert Abrams. His influence with the 'black box' referred to earlier was even stronger on the other side of the Atlantic than in Britain. As Gevitz (1988b) relates, he claimed that he could not only diagnose specific diseases from the vibrations they emitted, but also treat them using a device that would give off the same vibrations as the disease. The equipment was made available to physicians and others for leasing at several hundred dollars a month, on condition that the box that contained it was not opened. In his own medical career, Abrams had reached the exalted positions of President of the San Francisco Medico-Chirurgical Society and Vice-President of the California Medical Society. His high standing did not protect him from ridicule from the profession in the *Journal of the American Medical Association*. The 'black box' was also debunked in an investigation by a team including the Nobel Prize-winning physicist Robert Milliken. However, although the attack on such alternative practitioners within the profession was generally in line with medical self-interests at both élite and grassroots levels, the attention focused on Abrams by organized medicine seemed to backfire, as it fuelled popular demand for the device in the United States.

As in Britain, alternative practitioners defended their own position against medical orthodoxy, in line with their own interests. Rather than accepting the applicability of such terminology as 'quacks' and 'sects', they redefined themselves in their journals and other outlets as 'reformers' based on different 'philosophical schools' (Gevitz 1988b). They also referred to orthodox medicine as outdated, stressing that it was not so much their principles as those of the allopaths that were dogmatic. Alternative therapists such as chiropractors often presented themselves as being 'scientific' too – as opposed to medical orthodoxy, which they saw as being rooted in more speculative thinking (Wardwell 1992). At the same time, the value of their approach compared to that of orthodox medicine was emphasized, in terms of its greater safety and therapeutic benefit. Central to this claim were said to be the high rates of satisfaction of clients, even when physicians had previously unsuccessfully treated them (Gevitz 1988b). Such therapists defended the mental states of their patients – whose alleged credulity was seen as relating to conventional, not alternative, medicine. These arguments, based on similar selective stereotypes to those of medical orthodoxy, were reflected in the legal action that alternative practitioners took against state medical boards. For example, the osteopaths challenged them both for defining medicine too widely and for not licensing their own practice (Gevitz 1982).

State legislatures, nonetheless, sometimes backed alternative practitioners against organized medicine, despite the growing scientific legitimacy of the latter in the first half of the twentieth century. That they did so was in part testimony to the power of the ideology of alternative practitioners in the face of medical licensing laws that undermined the rights of citizens to decide for themselves in the health arena, and protected monopolistic medical interests. A particularly forceful case was made by the chiropractors with their campaign to 'go to jail for chiropractic', rather than pay the fines for illegal practice (Wardwell 1988). Ironically, some groups of alternative practitioners, such as osteopaths, sought legal protection themselves – and, in so doing, strove to combat 'imposters' and 'imitators'. For osteopaths at the beginning of the twentieth century these included chiropractors, whose training courses were less developed, as well as competitors with spurious qualifications (Gevitz 1988a). Thus in the United States at this time – as in Britain – occupational self-interests were not only being pursued by orthodox medicine.

Just as in the medical profession too, there were divisions within alternative practice itself. Internal debates over how far surgery and obstetrics should be included in the osteopathic curriculum (Gevitz 1982) and the extent to which 'straights' or 'mixers' should practise chiropractic in terms of its medical content (Wardwell 1976) illustrate this point. As on the other side of the Atlantic, such splits weakened lobbies for specific types of alternative medicine. Together with the perceived benefits of scientific research into conventional medicine, such divisions helped orthodox medicine increasingly to gain ascendancy over alternative medicine in the United States in the period up to the 1950s. This was underlined by the greater use made by the public of orthodox, as compared to unorthodox, practitioners (Gevitz 1988b).

The battle between the medical profession and the patent medicine manufacturers

Such ascendancy was also reflected in the outcome of the battle that took place between the medical establishment and commercial manufacturers of 'quack' remedies in the first half of the twentieth century, as in the British case. The challenge here came from the patent medicine manufacturers because they not only produced alternative remedies, but also gave general guidance on health and specific conditions to the public, which often conflicted with that provided by medical orthodoxy (Starr 1982). Their advertisements in the mass media undermined the authority of physicians because they usually explicitly or implicitly derided the work of doctors. As Burrow (1963) notes, they advocated remedies for a whole range of conditions, from tuberculosis and cancer to obesity and syphilis, most of which were branded as 'quackery'. The threat to the profession was thereby heightened, given the wide scale of employment of self-diagnosis and treatment in the United States at this time (Saks 2000a).

Although self-help was most widely used in areas where physicians were considered expensive and were not always readily available (Roebuck and Quan 1976), it is easy to understand from an interest viewpoint why the American Medical Association continued the campaign against patent medicine manufacturers that had been initiated in the previous century. As in Britain, the medical establishment strove to force them to disclose the secret formulas of their remedies. The *Journal of the American Medical Association* stopped publishing advertising for such preparations at the turn of the century and exhorted other medical journals, including the *British Medical Journal* (which had a less rigorous approach to advertising), to do the same (Bartrip 1990). Gevitz (1988b) says that it was hoped that such action would persuade lay periodicals and newspapers to follow suit. Although this strategy was not entirely successful – as the loss of revenue proved too much of a disincentive to many of the publications concerned – it illustrates another social control mechanism employed by the medical profession against unorthodox remedies. As Starr (1982) notes, this tactic was extended further when the American Medical Association later went on to forge an alliance with journalists campaigning against deceptive business practices, who took up the crusade against the lack of regulation of proprietary medicines as a major social issue. This crusade complemented the profession's own warnings about their hazards and underscored the need to consult a trained physician in the first instance from the viewpoint of public safety.

In terms of the interests of members of the profession who stood to lose business from such competition in a predominantly private, fee-for-service system, it was important that the battle was won against patent medicine manufacturers in forcing the disclosure of secret remedies. This indeed it was, as the medical profession grew in stature. The long and slippery slope for the companies involved in the first half of the twentieth century was marked first by the 1906 federal Pure Food and Drug Act. This formally banned false and fraudulent labels concerning the constituents of medicinal preparations, even if it did lack teeth (Burrow 1963). The main limitation of this Act was that it did not offer protection against products containing drugs with restricted utility, and could even have been construed by the public as providing government endorsement of the remedies concerned. The legislation was amended in 1912, though, to include fraudulent claims about effectiveness. Its scope was subsequently widened in the 1920s to apply to advertising in newspapers (Starr 1982). However, as Burrow (1963) observes, the Act was still not strongly enforced, with only two prison sentences being given within the first 30 years of its passage, despite thousands of violations.

The position changed, however, as the profession developed the finances to establish its own regulatory mechanism through the American Medical Association – which developed an approved list of products in 1907. The Council on Pharmacy and Chemistry, established to set standards for and test medicinal preparations, constructed the list. It excluded drugs for which the composition was not disclosed, as well as any product that was advertised to the public (Burrow 1963). The onus was on the importance of the public consulting physicians directly about medications, rather than stumbling upon remedies in the press. Many critiques of vendors of nostrums and their remedies were included in the *Journal of the American Medical Association*, ranging from attacks on their lack of effectiveness to criticism of their relatively high costs. These tactics were complemented by the production of two volumes by the American Medical Association (1912, 1921) entitled *Nostrums and Quackery*, which aimed to expose fraudulent remedies sold by the patent medicine manufacturers. As a result of these, many newspapers were finally persuaded to sacrifice advertising income in the interests of public health by refusing to publicize such products. Indeed, some states even legislated to prevent newspapers from carrying such advertisements (Starr 1982).

In the period between the wars, the American Medical Association set up a Bureau of Investigation to generate further evidence against commercial companies operating in this area (Burrow 1963). It continued to highlight 'quackery' and 'exploitation' in its journal and other publications, while still endeavouring to restrict advertising outlets for such preparations. The attempts of the Association to strengthen legislation for patent medicines finally led in 1938 to the federal Food, Drug and Cosmetic Act. This not only introduced more stringent requirements for the approval of new drugs and lengthened the list of potentially hazardous drugs that had to appear on the labels of relevant products, but also imposed heavier penalties for those who transgressed the rules. Although this did not stop the public from engaging in self-treatment, it stifled some of the demand for patent medicines. It also ensured that doctors had more direct control of purchasing decisions by consumers through the Act's strategic gatekeeping role, which was reinforced by its increasing association with science and was in the business interest of most physicians (Starr 1982).

Although some doctors supported the use of patent medicines, the medical profession in the United States was more cohesive in the first half of the twentieth century than first meets the eye. This cohesion helped it to advance its collective interests in terms of income, status and power by limiting the influence of the patent medicine manufacturers. However, the nostrum makers – just like unorthodox practitioners – fought back against the medical profession in a manner consistent with their own interests. Some sought damages through the courts. The vendors of the highly alcoholic Wine of Cardui for female ailments, for instance, brought a successful libel suit against the American Medical Association in 1916 for its charge that their business was 'built on deceit' (Burrow 1963). The patent medicine manufacturers often argued too that physicians were serving their own ends by attacking their cheap cures in order to charge high fees for more lengthy and expensive treatments. They also sometimes claimed to have endorsements from eminent physicians or to run a medical institute – or even to be doctors themselves – to legitimate their claims. In addition, they employed the terminology associated with the latest discoveries in medicine, as well as the increasing credibility of 'science' in American society at this time (Starr 1982).

The rising standing of medical practice ultimately led the patent medicine manufacturers to come to heel. As a result of growing federal regulation and lobbying by the American Medical Association, the companies placed greater emphasis on the importance of the patient consulting the physician in cases of serious illness (Starr 1982). They also gradually drew back from the wider panacea claims that they had made at the beginning of the century. Advertising standards across the health field were tightened too, as the use of unorthodox medicine was restricted (Burrow 1963). This paralleled the success of the medical profession in restraining alternative practice, which had led the numbers of homoeopaths significantly to decline by the 1950s (Kaufman 1988). In consequence, the attempt by the medical establishment to control alternative medicine in the first part of the twentieth century in the United States – as in Britain – had a real effect in diminishing its practice inside and outside medical orthodoxy. The profession was thereby able to restrict public opportunities to use the medical alternatives, inevitably generating greater inequalities of access (Saks 2000a).

The increasing medical incorporation of alternative medicine

However, here the similarity with Britain ends, for alternative medicine was at a conspicuously lower ebb there than in the United States by the mid-twentieth century. This was mainly because American physicians adopted a more incorporationist stance towards alternative medicine than their British counterparts as the middle of the century approached. There was, for example, more ready acceptance of acupuncture by doctors. Following on from the positive medical reception given to this therapy on both sides of the Atlantic in the early nineteenth century, limited medical interest in this procedure continued into the early twentieth century in the United States, unlike in Britain (Saks 1995b). The greater orthodox tendency to assimilate alternative practices was even more apparent from the growing *rapprochement* in the United States between osteopathy and the medical profession (Baer 1987). Although full incorporation had not occurred by the mid-twentieth century, from the 1930s onwards the curriculum of American osteopathic colleges started to follow that of orthodox medical schools. As Gevitz (1988a) notes, this, together with rising public demand for their services, led osteopaths to gain independent licensing rights in 38 states by the 1950s – as well as hospital privileges that extended their role. While the American Medical Association still referred to osteopathy as 'cultist healing' (Cohen 1998), its gradual assimilation served the interests of orthodox medicine by helping to resolve its internship shortage (Gevitz 1988a).

The cases of acupuncture and osteopathy in the United States highlight not only that incorporation in selected areas had taken place by the 1950s, but also that it was largely being conducted on the medical profession's own terms. The same was true of homoeopathy. Although, as we have seen, it was increasingly marginalized following its alliance with orthodox medicine at the turn of the century, there were signs that the relationship might once again be re-established. As Kaufman (1988) notes, the American Institute of Homoeopathy forged common cause with the American Medical Association over the threat posed by 'socialized medicine' in the Roosevelt years. It was possible in the 1940s that this might be built upon and lead to homoeopathy being accepted as an orthodox therapeutic specialty under the non-sectarian framework of a new Board of Homeotherapeutics. This could be seen as an interest-based incorporationist strategy, as specialist status would have reduced the challenge of the conflicting theoretical base of homoeopathy. However, the American Medical Association ultimately decided against this, after several years of discussion with the homoeopaths.

Although the medical incorporation of alternative therapies in the United States was more extensive than in Britain, it also had its limits. It had not developed by the mid-twentieth century quite as far as indicated by Moran and Wood (1993: 39) to include 'greater tolerance of the existence of chiropractors'. Despite the growing popularity of chiropractors, this occupational group and the American Medical Association were a long way from being happy bedfellows, in part because practitioners of chiropractic had a less substantial biomedical base than their counterparts in osteopathy (Baer 1987). When it could not stop it from being licensed in the United States, organized medicine instead sought to control chiropractic through state medical boards – with the tightest possible definition of its scope of practice. The trade-off for chiropractors in some states was a generous grandparent clause licensing existing chiropractors without the need for further examination (Wardwell 1988). Nonetheless, as we shall see in the following chapters, the general tendency was for alternative medicine to be increasingly assimilated into medical orthodoxy. This trend was more pronounced in the second half of the twentieth century in the United States, where fuller incorporation again occurred significantly more rapidly than in Britain.

The difference in the level of medical incorporation of alternative medicine in Britain and the United States in the period from the professionalization of medicine to the mid-twentieth century may be partly explained in terms of public demand in the more open, populist *laissez-faire* culture of the latter, a culture that made it more difficult to suppress unorthodox practices than in Britain (Saks 2000a). However, the key explanation of the variation in the response of the medical profession to alternative medicine from an interest-based neo-Weberian perspective seems to be the differential legal terms on which the exclusionary social closure of medicine was based. Crucial to this interpretation is the distinctive British common law that allowed anyone to become an alternative therapist, even without training – despite legislation restricting the scope of such practice (Larkin 1995). In this situation, it has typically not been in the interests of the medical élite to support the incorporation of unorthodox procedures, even in the face of public demand, because of the danger of legitimating outsiders. Doing so would threaten not only to create greater competition in the private sector, but also to subvert the monopoly rights of medicine – especially when a number of its rivals have longer experience of alternative medicine and subscribe to conflicting theories of medicine.

There have, of course, been occasions historically when the British medical profession has been prompted to incorporate alternative approaches in the face of external pressures. A good example is its moderation of the harsher aspects of the heroic therapies in the latter half of the nineteenth century in Britain in response to the challenge posed by the gentler approach of the homoeopaths (Nicholls 1988). Incorporation, though, was not generally an attractive option from the mid-nineteenth century onwards in terms of medical interests because of the nature of the regulatory arrangements underpinning professionalization. By contrast, in the United States in the first half of the twentieth century, concerns about competition from outsiders were reduced because occupational rivals were often not allowed to practise under the law in the state-based licensing system. As Larson (1977) suggests, the medical dominance of the licensing boards that were established enabled orthodox medicine to limit external competition. At the same time, it allowed the assimilation of the methods of competitors where this was compatible with maintaining or enhancing the income, status and power of the profession. In such circumstances, there was less risk of opening the floodgates to non-medical practitioners of alternative medicine through incorporation in the American licensing system, as compared to the British regulatory framework with its provisions for common law practice (Saks 1995b).

ACCOUNTING FOR THE MARGINALIZATION OF ALTERNATIVE MEDICINE IN BRITAIN AND THE UNITED STATES

The above account attempts to explain the variation in the response by organized medicine to unorthodox therapies in Britain and the United States from a neo-Weberian perspective with reference to the different forms of licensure in the societies concerned. It is not, however, without its complexities. It is predicated on the assumption that licensing laws were generally enforced in the period following the professionalization of medicine up to the mid-twentieth century, in contrast to much of the earlier period in the Anglo-American context (Berlant 1975). As will also be apparent from the foregoing discussion, the balance of medical interests ultimately needs to be judged in terms of particular forms of unorthodox therapy and cannot readily be applied to alternative medicine as a whole, given the diversity of the field. Thus the balance of medical interests in any specific case will depend on a broad range of influences. These include factors such as the level of demand for the therapy, the compatibility of its philosophies with biomedicine, the size and internal cohesiveness of the members of the group involved, and the level of grassroots medical employment of the therapy concerned (see, for instance, Baer 1987). Such interests, moreover, cannot be abstracted from the social, political and economic context of the health system and wider society in which they are embedded (Moran and Wood 1993).

The chapter concludes by focusing on the similarities rather than the differences in the medical response to unorthodox medicine in Britain and the United States – and particularly the common pattern of marginalization of alternative practice in both these countries. The emphasis here is on the reasons why the overarching climate was still, by the 1950s, primarily marked by the professional rejection of alternative medicine. Thus far it has been argued that the marginalization of unorthodox practices inside and outside the profession in the Anglo-American context can largely be explained in terms of the interests of doctors – as they endeavoured to sustain and, where possible, advance their income, status and power in the face of competition. The implementation of such interests at various levels was clearly facilitated by the powerful platform of exclusionary closure established through the professionalization of medicine on both sides of the Atlantic. This facilitative framework was enhanced by the growing unity of the medical profession, based on the biomedical paradigm, in the period up to the mid-twentieth century. Moreover, while some of its unorthodox rivals were men – such as the osteopaths (Gevitz 1982) – medical interests may also have been furthered by continuing male domination of the profession, which differentiated it from the female gender base of nursing and a number of other allied health professions in this period. This male domination may well have been important in consolidating its position in societies that remained patriarchal, despite a range of egalitarian social reforms (Witz 1992).

However, this neo-Weberian interpretation of the predominant medical rejection of unorthodox approaches to health care is contentious. It has been challenged by those who argue that the persisting medical marginalization of alternative therapies at this time was related not so much to professional self-interests, as to the protection of the health of the public. As was seen in the last chapter, a similar argument has been put forward by functionalist writers to explain the initial professionalization of medicine in the Anglo-American context. This argument is centred on the increasing capacity of scientific medicine to deal with disease following the bacteriological revolution, and the consequent need to stave off the threat of exploitation by the unqualified (Wallis and Morley 1976). As will be recalled, this claim was challenged on a variety of grounds, including the relative lack of effectiveness of orthodox medicine in the mid-nineteenth century in Britain and at the turn of the twentieth century in the United States. Had the position, though, sufficiently moved forward to counter the professional self-interest account of the predominantly negative medical response to alternative medicine in the period leading up to the mid-twentieth century?

There is no doubt, as was shown in Chapter 2, that biomedicine developed further on both sides of the Atlantic over this period. Its unified 'scientific' base certainly expanded as laboratory medicine came more fully on stream. Orthodox medicine also seems to have produced increasing practical pay-offs for the public, as many innovatory procedures were introduced – from the use of X-rays to the employment of penicillin (Dally 1997). While the medical profession was firmly in the ascendance by the 1950s, moreover, question marks were also raised about the comparative benefits of unorthodox medicine. In Britain the safety and utility of such alternative practitioners as the homoeopaths were regularly queried in the medical literature up to the mid-twentieth century, not least because of their potential to divert consumers from apparently more effective orthodox treatment (Nicholls 1988). Burrow (1963: 93) too sees the battle against groups such as the patent medicine manufacturers in the first few decades of the twentieth century in the United States in terms of the 'American Medical Association's struggle to protect the nation's health'. This is understandable when such manufacturers were urging adults and children to self-medicate with preparations containing unknown quantities of substances such as opium and alcohol in the early part of the century (Starr 1982).

The position, though, is again more complicated than it initially appears. This was still an age when effective remedies such as quinine were drawn from the unorthodox repertoire (Inglis 1980) and large numbers of technically needless operations such as tonsillectomies were carried out by medical practitioners (Turner 1995). Clearly, debates will continue about the comparative merits of the activities of the medical profession and its competitors at this time. Whether the effectiveness of modern medicine was more important than that of medical self-interests is also not necessarily pivotal in determining the reasons for the marginalization of alternative medicine. In this regard, Bartrip (1990) believes that there are three types of explanation of the stance of doctors towards unorthodox therapies following the professionalization of medicine. The first is the rhetorical view presented in the mainstream medical journals that the general climate of rejection of alternative medicine was perpetuated to prevent the public from being defrauded, injured or killed. A second is that doctors acted self-interestedly to gain from their monopolization of medical practice, to the disadvantage of the public. The third view – developed further at the collective level by Saks (1995b) – is that professional interests and the public good are not bound to conflict and can go hand in hand, with advantages to doctors as well as the public. Although the overall balance of health benefit to the consumer may have tilted more in the direction of orthodox medicine by the mid-twentieth century, this point demonstrates the breadth of applicability of the neo-Weberian professional self-interest account – which is not dependent on the creation of public detriment.

There are, of course, other theoretical perspectives that could also be applied to make sense of the continuing generally negative medical response to unorthodox medicine in the Anglo-American context by the 1950s. These include those of the Marxist writers considered in Chapter 2, who base their views on the class relations of capitalism. As indicated earlier, they are not particularly convincing in accounting for the initial professionalization of medicine in the Anglo-American context. They are even less persuasive in explaining the persisting general climate of rejection of alternative therapies in the period following the establishment of the medical profession. Their lack of persuasiveness can be illustrated by the work of Brown (1979), who suggests that the ongoing marginalization of alternative medicine in the United States occurred because capitalists controlled the development of scientific medicine and this was more resonant with their worldview than holistic unorthodox therapies. The weakness of this position has been exposed by Starr (1982: 227–8), who satirically notes that the enquirer indeed needs 'a deep appreciation of the fragility of capitalism to imagine that it might have been threatened by the persistence of homoeopathy'. He adds that further difficulties are posed by the fact that a number of 'the most enthusiastic believers in scientific medicine ... were socialists, who were outraged by the failure to extend its benefits to the working class'. He therefore concludes that: 'the legitimacy of capitalism rested on more ample foundations than the alleged ideological functions of medicine in focusing attention on bacteria rather than class interests.'

There are dangers, therefore, in overstating the significance of the Marxist account, which again allows too little scope for the independent actions of the medical profession. However, the influence of class interests on the interface between orthodox and alternative medicine should not be completely overlooked in the period up to the 1950s. As we have seen, corporate interests had a significant, if not a monolithic, impact on the house of medicine in Britain and the even more market-oriented, business-driven health care system of the United States at this time (Higgins 1988; Navarro 1986). In this respect, though, it should be remembered that commercial interests in the patent medicine industry drove much of the challenge from alternative medicine to the medical profession in the early years of its existence. But if this observation counters the Marxist perspective in this area, it is also true that the multinational pharmaceutical companies that were to emerge have provided far more support thereafter for orthodox biomedicine on both sides of the Atlantic (Doyal 1979; Bodenheimer 1985). Looking ahead too, the 1960s and 1970s witnessed the development of a counter-culture that shook public faith in the drugs produced by such companies and other forms of modern medicine. This further dilutes the claim that the overall marginality of alternative medicine in Britain and the United States was based on the superior effectiveness of orthodox biomedicine. With these thoughts in mind, it is to this more recent period that the book now turns.

CHAPTER 4

The development of a medical counter-culture

This chapter begins by charting the background to the emergence of a strong medical counter-culture in Britain and the United States that peaked from the mid-1960s to the mid-1970s. It first outlines the associated developments in orthodox and unorthodox medicine in these two societies following the mid-twentieth century, primarily centred on the 1950s and the 1960s. The chapter then looks in more detail at the various strands of the medical counter-culture that emerged, situating it in its wider social context. The impact of this period that was highly critical of medical orthodoxy and other establishment institutions is then considered, on the basis not only of the expansion of the power of the consumer and self-help in health care, but also – and most particularly – of the upsurge of public interest in alternative therapies. Finally, the chapter examines the reaction of medical orthodoxy to such counter-cultural developments, focusing on the response that it made to unorthodox therapies, which crystallized the spirit of the challenge posed to the medical profession at this time.

HEALTH CARE IN THE 1950s AND 1960s

In terms of orthodox medicine, the confidence born of the first half of the twentieth century based on 'scientific' progress continued into the 1950s and 1960s in both Britain and the United States. As Le Fanu (1999) highlights, many new drugs were brought into effective use in this period, largely as a result of increased understanding of their chemistry, with the dozen or so recommended drugs available to doctors of the 1930s extending to some two thousand by the 1960s. In the ferment of the pharmacological revolution, these ranged from streptomycin for tuberculosis to chlorpromazine and the anti-depressants in psychiatry. The concept of intensive care also became more prevalent, including the use of ventilators to provide an adequate oxygen supply to assist the recovery of patients. This was the time too when open-heart surgery, hip replacements and kidney transplantation, among a plethora of other innovations, were introduced (Duin and Sutcliffe 1992). These paved the way for what was probably the greatest technical achievement in surgery in this period – the first heart transplant in 1967, which presaged the start of a series of such operations before this procedure was more extensively perfected. This latter example epitomized the optimism associated with the expansion of orthodox medicine at this time and the recession of the boundaries of what was believed to be possible, in the wake of technological developments. While the full impact of these developments was to be felt in the 1970s and beyond (see Blume 2000), they are an important backdrop to the development of the medical counter-culture in the Anglo-American context.

ORTHODOX MEDICINE IN BRITAIN

In Britain, the 1950s and 1960s was the period when the National Health Service, introduced in 1948, was becoming more fully established.[1] As was noted in Chapter 2, the aim of the government was to introduce a more centralized, comprehensive state-funded health care delivery system – bringing the growing benefits of developments in health care to a wider public in a more egalitarian fashion (Butler and Vaile 1984). This it proceeded to do against the background of an administratively confused system based on a mix of national insurance and private practice that had existed for most of the first half of the twentieth century (Stacey 1988). The National Health Service, though, was to be primarily focused on orthodox rather than alternative medicine, as the former continued to trade on the halo of science. However, the disparate framework within which health care was organized before World War II – characterized by substantial inequalities in provision – was to be transcended by a more planned system (Allsop 1995a). This was centred on the principles of care free at the point of access and equal entitlement to use, even for those who ultimately chose to purchase health provision from the private sector. In managerial terms, the system involved an elaborate organizational structure based on the creation of Regional Hospital Boards, Hospital Management Committees, and Executive Councils administering the operation of general practices. These paralleled the local health authorities that ran community services (Levitt et al. 1995).

Unsurprisingly, this period was marked by a flurry of government reports making various recommendations designed to increase the unification of the National Health Service. The need for these arose primarily because health care was split into a tripartite structure – covering hospitals, general practice and community care – with few common boundaries to facilitate cooperative working (Kingdom 1996). The split led to fragmentation and inefficiency that impacted on the quality of services, especially since integrative health centres were only slowly introduced up until the late 1960s (Gabe and Calnan 1991). The first major reorganization of the National Health Service was not to come until 1974, in part because of the difficulties of achieving an appropriate compromise on how to increase the unity of the service between the leaders of the medical profession and other interested parties (Allsop 1995a). The creation of a new top-down structure based on the retention of Regional Health Authorities, which were given a more strategic role in relation to hospital and community health services, highlighted the flaws of the previous system. So too did the establishment of Area Health Authorities responsible for planning and providing health services, which were largely coterminous with local authorities and associated with one or more District Health Authorities. Alongside these changes, the arrangements for general practice were little changed – with Family Practitioner Committees taking over in name only from Executive Councils in managing general practitioners (Stacey 1988).

From a professional viewpoint, the position of medicine was enhanced from the mid-twentieth century onwards, particularly in the hospital sector, where specialists and consultants benefited the most financially from the establishment of the National Health Service. Their gains came as a result of a combination of factors, including pay mechanisms, conditions of service and the facility to undertake private practice within their contracts (Gill 1975). Although capital investment was limited, hospitals – and especially the more privileged teaching hospitals – attracted an increasing share of government health expenditure. In a period of economic growth that was soon accompanied by a hospital modernization and building programme, specialization was promoted as each hospital strove to benefit from developments in specialist areas of medicine (Allsop 1995a). The number of specialists and the range of specialties grew apace with technological development, with the emergence of new specialisms in fields such as gastroenterology and clinical pharmacology, and the expansion of existing specialties such as cardiology and psychiatry (Le Fanu 1999). This trend was increasingly reflected in the nature of undergraduate and postgraduate medical education, as recommended in the 1968 Todd Report, which advocated a wider and more flexible curriculum. The so-called Cogwheel Reports published in 1967, 1972 and 1974 further recommended that in practice settings, broad specialty-linked groupings be established to coordinate clinical and administrative work in the National Health Service (Levitt et al. 1995).

However, despite the Cogwheel Reports, evidence suggests that in the majority of cases consultants continued to make resource decisions with relatively little reference to other health professional groups (Allsop 1995a). If the fact that they did so highlights the dominance of hospital consultants, general practitioners remained at the other end of the medical pecking order – being considered within the profession to be of lower status than hospital specialists in this period (Gill 1975). In terms of the market, general practitioners were similarly placed to small shopkeepers as they continued to be self-employed outside the formal administrative structure of the National Health Service, but contracted to provide services to it (Stacey 1988). Moreover, while hospital doctors heavily drew upon the research funding that was increasingly available for scientific work from bodies such as the Medical Research Council (see, for example, Thomson 1973), the professional development of general practitioners stagnated, mainly because of their poor work situation (Gabe and Calnan 1991). Their power was also reduced by the fact that hospital doctors no longer needed to rely for their income on referrals from them in their salaried posts in the National Health Service (Forsyth 1966). Although this reduction in their power had an adverse effect on the position of family doctors, it was mitigated by the founding in 1952 of the College of General Practitioners, which sought to improve conditions in general practice and in 1967 became a Royal College (Stacey 1992).

There continued, therefore, to be divisions in the power possessed by different segments of the medical profession in Britain in the 1950s and 1960s. These are further exemplified by the even more marginalized position of public health physicians, who not only failed to achieve a fully integrated health service, but also came under government control soon after they gained recognition as a medical specialty (Gill 1975). Nonetheless, the growing number of doctors at this time generally remained in control of health care as a corporate body, in a manner underwritten by the state through the legislation underpinning the National Health Service (Berlant 1975). There were high levels of medical representation on such bodies as the Regional Hospital Boards and Hospital Management Committees – which added to the influence that they wielded through professional advisory channels (Klein 1989). Their position on these bodies complemented their control over key areas such as the medical curriculum and disciplinary procedures (Stacey 1992). Leading figures from the British Medical Association and the Royal Colleges, moreover, formed an even more cohesive and definable élite at this time, underlined by the nature and level of their involvement on the General Medical Council (Saks 1995b). The control exercised by medical practitioners in general and the medical élite in particular was accentuated by their continuing dominance over the rest of the orthodox health care labour force, which virtually doubled in size in the thirty years following the founding of the National Health Service (Allsop 1995a).

Of this labour force, nurses were by far the largest group. Their standing was elevated, not least by the Salmon Report in 1967, which recommended a division between senior nurse managers and others carrying out traditional nursing roles. However, while this established professional nursing equivalents to their medical and administrative counterparts in management, nurses remained in practice in a subordinated position similar to that of the other professions allied to medicine (Dingwall *et al.* 1988). Their inferior position was highlighted when the hierarchical orthodox health care division of labour was consolidated through the 1960 Professions Supplementary to Medicine Act, which, as we have seen, initially included chiropodists, dietitians, medical laboratory technicians, occupational therapists, physiotherapists, radiographers and remedial gymnasts – extending to orthoptists in 1966 (Larkin 1983). Although the medical profession opposed their state registration, the dominant position of medicine in the relationship was explicit in the very umbrella title that such professions were given, reinforced by the presence of medical representatives on their individual registration boards (Larkin 1993). Limited professions such as dentistry and optometry, moreover, remained enclosed within their own professional boundaries in the terms defined by Turner (1995). In their cases, the boundaries were underlined by the 1957 Dentists Act, which set up the General Dental Council as the sole statutory licensing and registration body, and the 1958 Opticians Act that established the General Optical Council and confined the prescribing and dispensing of spectacles to opticians (Levitt *et al.* 1995).

These professional groups were in various ways subject to the authority of doctors in the British context. These subordinated and limited professions, moreover, were in turn often themselves responsible for an ever-growing range of health care support workers operating outside the professional structure in the 1950s and 1960s (Levitt *et al.* 1995). This arrangement reinforced the authority not only of the medical profession, but also of the other subordinated professions, which continued to form the largest part of orthodox medicine. In this respect, consumers were only just beginning to gain a real voice in health care. Indeed, the introduction of Community Health Councils as formal public watchdogs occurred only with the reorganization of the National Health Service in 1974 (Allsop 1995a). The fact that it took so long highlights the very limited accountability of the orthodox health professions in general and medicine in particular in Britain in the two decades following the mid-twentieth century. This position paralleled to some degree the situation in United States at this time, where widespread community engagement in health care had still to become a reality (Starr 1982). However, there were other forces at work to make for differences as well as similarities in the American health care system.

ORTHODOX MEDICINE IN THE UNITED STATES

The most crucial difference between Britain and the United States was that the health care system in the latter remained predominantly privatized, unlike the National Health Service (Chandler 1996). This meant that while attempts were made to unify the health system in Britain in the 1950s and 1960s, health care in the United States was more decentralized and less coordinated in this period (Fry 1969). The cost-effectiveness of the system was therefore more open to challenge, not least because of the frequent duplication of expensive facilities in a competitive marketplace (Abel-Smith 1976). To be sure, the federal government continued to make a financial contribution in such fields as the control of communicable diseases, mental health, sanitation and the establishment of municipal hospitals. However, the public was not universally guaranteed the supply of medical care free or at a nominal charge at the point of access, as in Britain (Stevens 1983). Since orthodox health care was primarily centred on the principle of fee-for-service and health insurance, it was not available to all groups in the community. By the end of the 1950s, for example, only about two-thirds of the population had any kind of hospital insurance (Starr 1982). This led to inequalities in access to health care based in large part on the differential ability of the population to pay for such services, which increasingly became an issue for government as time wore on. Crucially, however, the means to overcome such inequalities, even in the 1960s, was not seen to be 'socialized medicine', so much as changes within the more market-oriented American health care system. This view was resonant with the greater emphasis given to self-help and the freedom of individual choice in the political culture of the United States (Saks 1995b).

As Starr (1982) relates, one major market development from the mid-twentieth century onwards that helped to ameliorate inequalities of access to health care in America was the expanding numbers of employees who gained health benefits. These were provided through a range of mechanisms from the direct delivery of company medical services to incorporation in broader health plans. Unions were increasingly involved in agreeing such packages with managers for groups of workers. In this respect, they played an important role in the development of pre-paid group practice plans – which also included at this time popular independent initiatives such as the Kaiser-Permanente and Health Insurance Plans. These paralleled the growth on a smaller scale of the more substantial commercial insurance schemes, the numbers of subscribers to which overtook the non-profit Blue Cross and Blue Shield plans, which were sponsored by physicians and the hospitals. Such commercial policies in turn were increasingly based on group insurance. In consequence, by the late 1950s some 78 per cent of American families where the main earner was fully employed had health insurance. Although this still left significant gaps, it did represent progress in combating the great health inequalities that existed at this time (Stevens 1971).

So too did the introduction by the government in the mid-1960s of Medicare and Medicaid, which enhanced access for less privileged groups without challenging the mainstream principles on which health care was based in the United States (Aday *et al.* 1980). In this regard, the federally financed Medicare programme provided health insurance for the elderly, the eligibility and benefits for which were derived from national standards. Medicaid, on the other hand, was directed towards providing health care for the poor in receipt of welfare benefits, the provision for which could be varied by individual states (Moran and Wood 1993). Even here, though, the coverage was not comprehensive, and significant inequalities in access to health care persisted after the mid-1960s. While these were predominantly class-based, they also had other, interrelated dimensions, including those linked to rural locations and inner-city practice (Anderson 1989) – as well as ethnic minorities (Weiss 1997). By the 1970s, moreover, women still made up only approximately one in ten of medical students in the United States, as compared to some one in three in Britain (Leeson and Gray 1978). It was ironic that such health inequalities continued at a time when American health care expenditure was rising much more steeply than spending in the British National Health Service. It grew between five- and sixfold over the 20-year period under consideration, before the need to contain the mushrooming cost of health care became more fully appreciated. The growth reflected factors such as rising prosperity, the expansion of private health plans and increasing faith by the government in developments in medical science (Starr 1982).

As part of this trend, as Stevens (1971) notes, specialization expanded further in the 1950s and 1960s, with increasing numbers of doctors becoming full-time specialists, most commonly in surgery. Psychiatry was also favoured, with rising interest in such fields as alcoholism and drug addiction. Research funding in this and other key specialist areas continued to expand very rapidly under the sway of the ideology of 'scientific' medicine. This expansion primarily took place through the foundations and the National Institutes of Health, despite allegations of financial impropriety at this time in relation to the expenditure of some research grants. Specialization was more strongly mirrored in graduate medical education too, where the numbers of students planning to go into general practice declined. General practice, though, was not simply a poor relation in terms of income, status and power, as in Britain. Notwithstanding the formation of the American Board of Family Practice in 1969, there was a lack of balance in the health care system itself between secondary and primary care – the latter of which was not very visible

(Chandler 1996). The large amount of funding for the construction of hospitals under the state-administered Hill–Burton programme highlights the emphasis on the expansion of the secondary, at the expense of the primary, sector (Anderson 1989). This was further underlined by the 1974 National Health Planning and Resource Development Act, which established state control over the supply and quality of hospital beds. Although there was greater government support for an increasing move to community care through neighbourhood and mental health centres from the 1960s onwards, this move was not backed with federal resources in the same way as the expansion of hospital services (Starr 1982).

Another trend associated with medicine in the United States at this time was the significant constraint that the American Medical Association imposed on the supply of physicians through medical education in the 1950s, in the face of rising demand for orthodox health care. Its position contrasted with that taken by the medical profession in Britain. Friedman (1962) argues that the effect of restricting supply was that the income of physicians was driven up in the marketplace – particularly in highly rewarded specialist areas of hospital medicine – in the interests of members of the profession, rather than the consumer. However, the numbers of medical students did expand in the following decade – as the proportion of specialists in the profession rose to more than three-quarters of all medical practitioners by the late 1960s (Krause 1996). Large increases in the income of medical schools and a commensurate rise in their staffing accompanied this growth (Starr 1982). Professional self-interest also provides a helpful explanation of the large differences in doctor–patient ratios between specific American states in this period. These were greater than comparable geographical variations in Britain, and more closely correlated to states' economic and social attractiveness than to the incidence of ill health (Roemer 1977). These trends together testify to the influence of the medical profession in American society in the 1950s and 1960s. The power of the profession was also indicated by the considerable discretion that government support for health care in areas such as medical research, mental health and hospital construction typically left in the hands of physicians and other medical bodies.

Thus, professional autonomy was protected in Medicare. Although its introduction was strongly opposed by many physicians (see, for example, Colombotos 1969), it did not reduce medical independence as anticipated. The medical profession gained, as Medicare expanded the funding available to cover medical fees, while giving doctors considerable freedom over prescription, treatment and the cost of their services (Stevens 1971). Public support for health care, therefore, was not usually accompanied by public control over physicians in the period immediately following the mid-twentieth century.

Internal as well as external mechanisms for enforcing medical authority were also in place. The professorial 'chairman-chiefs' of medical schools and teaching hospitals were very powerful here. Covering much of the metropolis, they controlled policy-making in their areas of authority, as well as the careers of their medical charges (Starr 1982). The medical profession, however, was not omnipotent, even at this stage. Aside from growing intervention by the state, its lack of complete control is demonstrated by its acceptance of the need to coexist with the growing numbers of pre-paid group practice schemes, which as a result of legal judgments threatened to expand lay control of its activities. Despite the rise in membership of the American Medical Association to a high of 73 per cent in 1963, the profession was also increasingly subject to the broader power of private corporations in health care (Krause 1996). This trend was more conspicuous in the predominantly privatized American health care system than in the more strongly collectivized British health service.

As in Britain, the profession in the United States too came under challenge from the rapidly expanding health work force, precipitated by the knowledge that the numbers of health personnel in the mid-twentieth century would not be sufficient to meet the growing demand for health care. The scale of growth of this sector was such that from 1950 to 1970 the numbers of health workers grew even more dramatically than in Britain, from 1 million to some 4 million. Training schools for professions such as pharmacy, nursing and other paramedical occupations were increasingly established in this period alongside medical and dental schools (Starr 1982). Nursing registration by now required successful completion of basic courses spanning from 1 and 2 years for lower grades to degrees and higher degrees for those in more senior positions (Chandler 1996). Nor was specialization a prerogative of the medical profession, as the case of nursing also illustrates – as a range of specialisms from intensive care to coronary care nursing emerged with the development of 'scientific' medicine (Kalisch and Kalisch 1995). Although solo private practice still remained the dominant form of medical work at this time, there were approximately four health professionals to each physician (Stevens 1971) – which grew to only one doctor to every thirteen health workers by 1970, as in Britain (Larkin 2000). However, despite the potential threat from competitors inside orthodoxy, the medical profession continued to use its power over other health professions by generally ensuring that state licensure was granted only under medical supervision or in restricted fields of health care (Krause 1996).

By the 1970s, as Larkin (2000) observes, the American Medical Association and the American Hospital Association recognized in these terms 23 different allied health professions through their Allied Health Accreditation programme. At the same time, the American Society of Allied Health Professions, which was founded in 1967 to promote the standing and education of practitioners following the 1966 Allied Health Professions Personnel Training Act, included 139 occupations in its list of recognized college training programmes. While inclusion on the list helped to enhance the status and training of the groups concerned, it also perpetuated their subordination and limitation along the lines set out by Turner (1995), paralleling the position in Britain after the mid-twentieth century. The processes involved also sometimes led to interest-based struggles between such groups and the medical profession, as highlighted by the case of optometrists, with whom the American Medical Association sustained its long-running dispute over who had the authority to treat eye diseases. In a similar vein, there was also a legal battle at the beginning of the 1970s between the American Medical Association and the American Society of Medical Technologists, as members of the latter increasingly sought to see patients without medical referral (Larkin 2000). Such health professions as nursing in turn continued to develop their own hierarchical control over the non-professionalized labour force (Kalisch and Kalisch 1995). But if this provides some insight into the division of labour within medical orthodoxy following the mid-twentieth century, where did alternative medicine stand in this period in Britain and the United States?

ALTERNATIVE MEDICINE IN BRITAIN

In Britain alternative medicine remained in a comparatively weak position, as the National Health Service – from which it was excluded except in orthodox hands – gradually developed. Its growth limited the market for alternative therapies, which were primarily available only in the relatively small private sector. However, there were signs that alternative medicine was rising from its slumbers, as public interest slowly increased (Saks 1996). Until the 1960s, though, the medical élite managed to hold back its development – despite the growing establishment of more systematic courses in such areas as acupuncture for non-medical practitioners (Fulder 1996). The British medical establishment made only minor concessions to unorthodox medicine. One such case was the agreement of the Royal Colleges to become members – along with the major church denominations, hospital chaplaincy organizations and healing groups – of the Churches' Council for Health and Healing, which had been formed in the 1940s to foster the healing ministry (Saks 1999a). This body prompted an investigation by the British Medical Association into spiritual healing which reported in 1955. The report broadly agreed with a committee that the British Medical Association had established after World War I on this subject, which had concluded that any effective healing that took place could only be for functional disorders with a psychiatric origin, based on the power of suggestion. Claims of cures of organic disorders were accordingly rejected (Inglis 1980).

In general terms, then, alternative therapists continued to be rebuffed, particularly where they threatened to encroach on the medical market for patients. Fulder (1996) notes that the osteopaths were told in 1957 that they were not to be included in the Professions Supplementary to Medicine legislation, even though this would have given them a subordinate standing to medicine through the medical referral system. In 1963 they were informed that they would not be considered for independent registration without a consensus between the medical profession, the public and the Department of Health. This snub was not specific to the osteopaths, who probably had the strongest affinity with orthodox medicine of all the unorthodox practitioners. The chiropractors were to be similarly rejected when they applied to join the professions supplementary to medicine in the 1970s (Fulder and Monro 1981). This negative response to the attempts by such groups to join the exclusive club of medical orthodoxy was coupled with an escalating campaign against 'quackery' in the medical journals that was designed to restrict informal referrals from doctors to alternative therapists. This campaign complemented the formal ethical prohibitions still in force on associations with such practitioners (Saks 1996).

Nonetheless, the medical establishment was not always successful in imposing restrictions on unorthodox medicine. For example, the British Medical Association was unable to persuade the Ministry of Health to stop spiritual healers from visiting patients who asked for their services in National Health Service hospitals in the 1950s and 1960s. This was despite the appearance of an editorial in the *British Medical Journal* that claimed such 'magical' healing was 'a return to the cave' and flew in the face of the achievements of 'scientific' medicine (Inglis 1980). However, at this time the exclusionary strategy of medical orthodoxy was generally effective in marginalizing alternative practice both inside and outside the profession. It was implemented through the controls that the medical élite maintained on, among other things, entry to medical school, the medical curriculum, and the growing amounts of funding for medical research. At a local level too, the boundaries of acceptability were marked by the blocking of unorthodox research proposals by local medical committees and the stigma that alternative therapies carried in medical circles. The influence of the latter was so great that even by the early 1970s, doctors belonging to the Scientific and Medical Network, a body of experts set up to explore fringe knowledge, wished to avoid their identities being publicized (Saks 1996). Significant changes, however, eventually took place in the wake of the development of the strong medical counter-culture in Britain from the mid-1960s onwards.

ALTERNATIVE MEDICINE IN THE UNITED STATES

A similar situation existed in the United States in relation to alternative medicine in the 1950s and 1960s. Here, it will be recalled, alternative therapies were generally in a stronger position than in Britain by the mid-twentieth century. The medical profession, though, broadly maintained its control over the next two decades – even if it was in its interests selectively to incorporate some therapies, as the counter-culture emerged. For example, osteopaths by then had rights and privileges similar to those of physicians in most states. Their case was helped by the fact that their work was partly underpinned by medical training. Indeed, when an American Medical Association committee investigated osteopathic training schools in 1959, it concluded that their standards of entry and qualification were at least as high as those of orthodox medical schools (Inglis 1980). Their high standards should not be too surprising as since 1951 they had been receiving federal support normally designated only for medical and dental colleges (Gevitz 1988a). Although this support raised issues about the distinctive identity of osteopaths, a further important symbolic event in the development of osteopathy was the merger in the early 1960s of the California Medical Association and the California Osteopathic Association. With the rising number of state-sponsored osteopathic colleges and state licensing arrangements making osteopaths the equals of physicians, they had largely become professionally incorporated into orthodox medicine in the United States by the early 1970s – unlike in Britain at a parallel stage of development (Baer 1987).

Chiropractors were a little further behind in terms of legitimacy, although by the 1960s chiropractic was recognized in most American states and in the early 1970s even received a small amount of federal research funding (Wardwell 1988). Moreover, where they practised medicine without a licence or illegally dispensed drugs, sympathetic juries frequently would not convict them – especially in areas that were underpopulated by physicians (Inglis 1980). This public sympathy highlights the growing strength of alternative medicine in the United States at this time, which is also indicated by the case of the homoeopaths. Despite the switchback ride that the homoeopaths experienced at the hands of the medical profession in the first half of the twentieth century, they finally achieved occupational unity by the 1950s when the International Hahnemannian Association and the more eclectic American Institute of Homoeopathy came together (Kaufman 1988). Homoeopathic licensing boards were also established in some states. Some chiropractors at this time even endeavoured to form 'homoeopathic colleges' to produce legitimate practitioners through such a licensing board in the state of Maryland. These attempts inevitably created tensions within unorthodoxy itself, which illustrates the weaknesses of alternative medicine as a lobby in relation to the power of the more unified American Medical Association. This latter body drew this practice to the attention of both the homoeopaths and the state authorities, in order that legal action could be taken.

Continuing divisions in this field also persisted between the osteopaths and chiropractors, groups who had different identities in spite of their superficially overlapping functions (Gevitz 1988a). However, the solidarity of unorthodox practitioners remained important in the 1950s and 1960s, notwithstanding increasingly favourable public opinion about alternative therapies – even if this solidarity was only within specific occupational boundaries. The need for it is underlined by the sustained attack on chiropractors by the medical establishment in this period, as illustrated by the establishment of the Committee on Quackery by the American Medical Association in 1971, which aimed, among other things, to first contain and then eliminate chiropractic. As a result, chiropractors were faced with the reluctance of third-party payers to cover treatment by themselves and other alternative therapists. This problem was exacerbated by the introduction of Medicare, in which chiropractic was not included until 1972 (Wardwell 1988). The need for greater unity in the face of potential adversity was also demonstrated by amendments in 1962 to the Pure Food and Drug Act that meant that the Food and Drug Administration had to ensure the effectiveness of all drugs on the market. Herbalists were early victims of its subsequent vigorous attack on 'health quackery' (Griggs 1997), although it initially focused on prescription drugs. The switch to over-the-counter medications from the early 1970s, however, created turmoil among homoeopaths because of fears about the standard against which its remedies would be evaluated. While this was eventually resolved by excluding homoeopathic remedies from the review, the issue was to resurface in heightened form a decade later (Kaufman 1988).

These adversarial encounters between orthodox and alternative medicine in both Britain and the United States were the precursor to a significant change of climate, as a strong counter-culture developed in the Anglo-American context from the latter half of the 1960s onwards. Ironically, the state of technological sophistication of orthodox medicine had never been greater in either Britain or the United States (Blume 2000). Against this, however, growing orthodox medical faith in the ability of high-technology medicine to deal with every malaise of humankind on the basis of 'scientific' progress – through revolutions in drugs and surgery and other technological innovations – was beginning to look increasingly tenuous. It was against this background that the medical counter-culture emerged across the Western world in general – and in Britain and the United States in particular. It formed part of a wider wave of disaffection in relation to the established order.

THE NATURE OF THE EMERGING MEDICAL
COUNTER-CULTURE

THE CONCEPT OF THE MEDICAL COUNTER-CULTURE

The concept of the medical 'counter-culture' in this context is defined as a subculture set up in opposition to the dominant culture of medicine. In this sense, at an abstract level, the nature of the 'counter-culture', just like that of 'alternative medicine' itself, varies historically and internationally according to the dominant orthodoxy in any particular society (Saks 2000a). In the case of Britain and the United States, this orthodoxy by the 1960s was most certainly based on biomedicine. The 'counter-culture' was not unique at this time. It had in effect existed since the professionalization of medicine in the mid-nineteenth century in Britain and the start of the twentieth century in the United States. Its existence is exemplified by the trends in the use of alternative medicine in these two countries, as described in Chapter 3 and in the first part of this chapter. There were a number of pockets in the community up to the middle of the twentieth century too where orthodox medicine was not normally used by the public at all. These included areas where doctors were either unavailable or did not meet the expressed needs of ethnic minority groups (see Roebuck and Quan 1976; Jones 1994). A broader illustration of the counter-culture is also contained in the early twentieth-century play *The Doctor's Dilemma* by George Bernard Shaw (1975), in which the medical profession and other kindred professions are depicted as 'conspiracies against the laity'.

Although there had been an undercurrent of public scepticism about medical orthodoxy since its establishment in both Britain and the United States, what was different about the mid-1960s was the scale and intensity with which this was manifested. The emergence of a strong medical counter-culture was also importantly associated with the wider social changes that were taking place in the West. As Roszak (1970) observes, the long-standing materialistic values that emphasized the delivery of technocratic solutions to problems generally came under fire at this time. The ideology of 'scientific progress' was also debunked, as growing numbers of the public sought to escape from established patterns of deference to authority and to explore alternative lifestyles. In striving to overcome the perceived spiritual vacuum in the 'scientific' age, new departures were taken in many areas of life – from fashions in clothes and hairstyles to the taking of hallucinogenic drugs such as LSD. Meditation and mysticism came to the fore, driven by the yearning for a more 'natural' existence and an expanding interest in Eastern philosophies

(Saks 1997b). An essential part of the general counter-culture that developed from this social critique on both sides of the Atlantic was also the increasing questioning of professional experts, including doctors – as well as groups such as architects and lawyers (Saks 2000a).

This growing challenge in the health arena drew on the early work of René Dubos (1959: 1), who warned of 'medical utopias' and the 'mirage of health' by noting that whatever progress is made in medical research, 'complete freedom from disease ... is almost incompatible with the process of living'. Following on from this, orthodox medicine came under particular attack in the 1960s for its lack of effectiveness, for creating doctor-induced disease, and for dehumanizing the patient. The main initial target was institutional psychiatry, which was seen by anti-psychiatrists as an instrument of therapeutic oppression dealing with the mythical condition of 'mental illness' (see, for instance, Szasz 1970; Laing 1976). The critique soon took on broader dimensions as it shifted to highlight a wider range of catastrophic effects of medical interventions, from the consequences of the routine prescription of thalidomide to pregnant women to the equivocal results produced by mutilating radical surgery for breast cancer (see, for example, Pietroni 1991). Critics also used epidemiology to underline that most of the advances in health since the nineteenth century were related to such factors as improved diet and sanitation, rather than biomedical intervention (McKeown 1979). This attack was crystallized by Ivan Illich (1976), who drew on a welter of contemporary evidence to argue that modern Western medicine had now become counterproductive. While it had initially brought some benefit, he claimed that – in striving unrealistically to chase the goal of immortality – high-technology medicine had created a modern nemesis by passing through a watershed that made it a positive threat to health.

THE CONSUMER, SELF-HELP AND THE MEDICAL COUNTER-CULTURE

Although issue can be taken with the one-sided nature of the arguments of Illich and other critics in this period (see, for instance, Bunker 1997), there is no doubt that they captured the spirit of the time. In the health arena, they signalled the development of the power of the consumer in Britain and the United States. In this respect, the counter-culture provided a platform for patients to exert rising pressure for greater professional accountability in orthodox medicine. In Britain the role of the consumer in health care has since been increasingly recognized in representational roles both on professional regulatory bodies and within key committees in the National Health Service.

Consequently, more data have become available about health options and the standards of health care to inform consumer choice. Consumers have also increasingly used the courts to win their rights (Allsop 1995a). In the United States litigation has proved an even more powerful tool for enhancing the accountability of the medical profession to the consumer. It was particularly effectively employed in the health rights movement that developed from the late 1960s onwards. This movement importantly strove to obtain not only rights to health care for the public, but also rights in relation to issues such as informed consent, the refusal of treatment, and access to personal records (Starr 1982).

Public criticism of medical orthodoxy linked to the emergence of a strengthened counter-culture has predictably tended to be greatest in areas where orthodoxy has least to offer or there are significant social concerns – such as chronic disorders, disability and organ transplantation (Williams and Calnan 1996). Lay subcultures with health philosophies that conflict with orthodox biomedicine have also contributed to the challenge to orthodox health care (Helman 2000). The informal social networks on which they are based can heavily influence the interpretation of symptoms and treatment decisions, including compliance with the advice of health professionals and self-prescription (Britten 1996). In this latter respect, self-help has played a fashionable part in recent developments involving the consumer in the health arena, frequently going beyond the boundaries of the traditional doctor–patient relationship as conceived from a biomedical perspective (Salmon 1985). It should be stressed, though, that self-help cannot always legitimately be seen as a counter-cultural phenomenon as it can operate within orthodox parameters, without challenging professional power. However, it becomes one when self-help activity represents resistance to the dominance of orthodox medicine, striking against mainstream values and institutions in health care – often through the vehicle of small-scale, non-hierarchical, participative organizational forms (Vincent 1992).

In this sense, self-help was central to the medical counter-culture that emerged in the 1960s and 1970s. At a collective level, the self-help tradition paved the way for a large number of groups campaigning for user interests, from those concerned with the health of black people to campaigns on HIV/AIDS. Examples of these range from the Patients Association in Britain to the National Women's Health Network in the United States (Saks 2000a). The part played by the women's movement has been particularly significant in health developments in the Anglo-American context. Initially, it focused its critique on the sexist treatment of women as consumers of orthodox health care, while lamenting the low proportion of female doctors and medical students (Stacey 1985). In Britain, it has now switched to such tasks as defending the role of Well Women Clinics in the state-financed health system and advancing the general living and working conditions of women. In the more privatized framework of the United States, meanwhile, the main feminist emphasis has been on establishing alternative health care provision for women that minimizes the role played by orthodox health professionals (Kelleher *et al*. 1994). In so doing, it has built on the work undertaken from the 1960s onwards by groups such as the Chicago Women's Liberation Union, which was distinguished by its underground abortion referral service. It has also benefited from the activity of the Boston Women's Health Collective, which played a high-profile role in demedicalization, by lobbying and providing counter-information for women on subjects such as home birth (Phillips and Rakusen 1989).

Other counter-cultural action since the 1970s in the self-help field has ranged from lay challenges to medical definitions of public and environmental health in legal disputes over leukaemia (Williams and Popay 1994) to anti-vivisectionist animal rights activity to prevent animals from being employed in medical research (Elston 1994). As we have seen, such activity has not only reinforced the radical consumer lobby, but also facilitated greater local self-provision of health care and advice, echoing the predominant form of health care in the pre-industrial past. The social networks in which self-responsibility for health is situated have been increasingly broadened too to include national and international dimensions in recent years, through the provision of health information in the mass media – not least via the expanding use of the Internet (Valente 2000). In North America and Western Europe the growing trend to take on self-responsibility for health has covered everything from the widespread purchase of stationary exercise cycles to enhance personal fitness to annual efforts by large numbers of smokers to desist from their habit to improve their health (Goldstein 2000). Although such types of self-help have not necessarily radically challenged the medical establishment in themselves, they can be loosely linked to the counter-culture of the 1960s and 1970s in so far as they depart from the conventional biomedical objectification of the patient in addressing issues of health and illness.

As Saks (1998a) notes, where such self-help activity falls under the strict definition of being counter-cultural, it may be seen as a philosophical departure from the modernist conception of health with which biomedicine is aligned. The notion of 'modernity' here is variously associated with grand theories, large-scale bureaucratic forms, regulation and surveillance, materialistic values, the notion of rational progress, complex bodies of objective knowledge, and the central role of the expert (see, for instance, Hall *et al*. 1992). In these terms, it is highly resonant with the development of orthodox biomedicine outlined in this book, including its rise to dominance through the professionalization of medicine. In contrast, the self-help element of the counter-culture has stronger affinities with the concept of 'postmodernity', based on fragmentation, local determination, a plurality of cultures, tolerance of diversity, multiple discourses, the denial of absolute knowledge, and the centrality of consumer choice (see, for example, Bertens 1995). Of course, there are major debates about whether modernity has been transcended at a societal level (Giddens 1991) – and whether the wide range of health and other forms that emerged in the 1960s and 1970s represent a move towards postmodernity (Coward 1989). Nonetheless, the polar types of modernity and postmodernity provide a framework within which the ideological basis of the substantial medical counter-culture that has emerged on both sides of the Atlantic can be analysed.

THE GROWTH OF ALTERNATIVE MEDICINE AND THE MEDICAL COUNTER-CULTURE

The strongest consumer-led counter-cultural development in health stemming from the mid-1960s in Britain and the United States was the rising public interest in the diverse array of alternative therapies that spread to most of the Western world over this period (see, *inter alia*, Clarke 1990; Lewith and Aldridge 1991). This certainly appears to represent a shift in the direction of postmodernity. In the Anglo-American context, the take-up of such therapies increased from a limited base in the first half of the twentieth century to a far more significant level. It is estimated in Britain that between one-fifth and one-third of the population have now used alternative medicine at some point (Fulder 1996), a similar range to that found in most of the rest of Europe (Fisher and Ward 1994). In the United States, meanwhile, survey evidence shows that the proportion of the public now using unorthodox medicine has risen from one-third (Eisenberg *et al.* 1993) to two-fifths (Eisenberg *et al.* 1998). This rise parallels the current relatively high utilization rate of alternative medicine in Canada in the North American context (Kelner and Wellman 1997a). This trend is not dissociated from the growth in self-help activity linked to the counter-culture, as many of the alternative therapies concerned – including aromatherapy and reflexology – are also employed on a self-help basis (Saks 2000a). In this respect, a large amount of the present use of alternative medicine has been centred on the fast-expanding sales of over-the-counter health foods and remedies (Bakx 1991).

That said, much of the spiralling demand by the public has been for practitioners of the more popular alternative therapies, such as acupuncturists, homoeopaths and herbalists. In Britain about one in seven of the population

visits an alternative practitioner for treatment each year (Sharma 1995), while
in the United States this figure is currently closer to one in five (Eisenberg *et al.*
1998). The numbers of non-medical practitioners of such therapies have also
grown alongside the increasing demand. In the early 1980s in the United
Kingdom there were estimated to be thirty thousand alternative therapists, of
whom the largest group were healers (Fulder and Monro 1981). A decade and
a half later the number had increased to forty-five thousand (Mills and
Peacock 1997), with the latest figure now being sixty thousand practitioners
(Mills and Budd 2000). The prevalence of alternative therapists in Britain,
though, is dwarfed by the scale of the practice of unorthodox medicine in the
far more populous United States, where the number of chiropractors alone
now rivals that of all such practitioners on the other side of the Atlantic
(Wardwell 1994a). In both countries, though, the numbers of alternative
practitioners outstrip those of general medical practitioners by a considerable
margin (Fulder 1996; Eisenberg *et al.* 1998). This comparison is distorted by
such factors as the part-time status of many alternative practitioners in Britain
and the decline of the generalist in the delivery of health care in the United
States. However, it does starkly highlight the contemporary significance of
unorthodox medicine in the Anglo-American context.

Despite rising public demand in Britain, such practice has remained
predominantly located in the private sector. This is a major point of
contention because although alternative therapists spend much more time
with patients than general practitioners (Fulder 1996), there may be major
cost savings associated with some types of alternative medicine in
comparison with high-technology medicine (Saks 1994). A MORI poll in
the late 1980s, moreover, indicated that some three-quarters of the
population wished to have more established alternative therapies included
in the National Health Service. While such a development has not yet fully
occurred, the Secretary of State for Health in 1991 for the first time clarified
that there was no government objection in principle to alternative medicine
being subcontracted out in the state sector (Saks 1991a). This statement
represented a significant change of position from that of the 1980s. At that
time the government had placed exacting requirements on alternative
therapists for them to gain a greater foothold in the National Health Service.
More specifically, it unrealistically expected that a unified case needed to be
presented on behalf of all alternative therapists if consideration were to be
given to enhancing their statutory position in the health sector (Sharma
1995). In the more privatized American health care system, public pressure
has contributed to some robust forms of alternative medicine being covered
by health insurance schemes in many states (Bruce and McIlwain 1998).
Inclusion in such schemes has helped to offset the costs that consumers

incurred for such therapies on a fee-for-service basis – thus increasing public access to alternative medicine (Taylor 1985).

There are, therefore, differences as well as similarities in the availability of unorthodox medicine, partly related to variations in the financial structure of the health systems in Britain and the United States. Following the mid-1960s there have also been contrasts between the two systems in the popularity of particular types of alternative medicine. Thus, in Britain osteopathy has generally found much more public favour than chiropractic, whereas the position is reversed in the United States (Baer 1987). At a generic level, it is often assumed that the growth of consumer interest in unorthodox medicine has largely taken place because of a revolutionary shift towards 'new age' values linked to the development of the counter-culture. These values are typically held to include the desire by the public for holistic health and greater participation in health care (Bakx 1991). To be sure, some of those who use such therapies do so because they conceive of health in terms of the whole person and wish to enhance control over their own being – avoiding the counter-productive effects of mainstream medicine in the process. Sometimes, too, such users possess a worldview based on subcultural values such as feminism, with a focus on their inner lives (Astin 2000; Furnham and Vincent 2000). Despite this link with the medical counter-culture, though, members of the public who employ alternative therapies in Britain and the United States have tended not to use them to the exclusion of orthodox medicine – however critical they may be of the latter (Thomas *et al.* 1991; McGuire 1988). In practice, consumers usually turn to such therapies for a restricted span of conditions and make pragmatic judgements as to the relative benefits of biomedicine and alternative medicine, when the former is not producing the desired results (Saks 2001).

Consumers, however, are not necessarily well informed about the benefits or otherwise of alternative therapies, even within the supportive framework of the social networks in which they are embedded (Valente 2000). This is especially so given the wide range of therapies that are encompassed by the notion of alternative medicine. Contrary to popular opinion, they can carry significant risks to health – despite their frequent ideological association with the safety of a 'natural' approach to health care (Ernst 2000). Herbal remedies such as sage and parsley, for instance, can cause abortion and haemorrhaging respectively (Eagle 1978), while the much-publicized cancer preparation laetrile has been found to be potentially lethal as it contains cyanide (Weiss 1997). The practice of acupuncture has led to a range of hazards, from collapsed lungs to hepatitis B (Macdonald 1982). Negative effects, though, seem to be reported relatively rarely (Fulder 1996). In terms of safety, the risks involved have for long tended to be more than counterbalanced by the dangers posed by orthodox medicine, including those arising from the routine administration of treatments such as chemotherapy, radiotherapy and surgery for cancer and other prevalent conditions (Berliner 1985b). To add to the dilemmas of consumers in making informed choices in relation to their own well-being, important issues have also been raised about the efficacy of alternative medicine.

In terms of efficacy, the main difficulty is that there have been relatively few rigorously conducted randomized controlled trials of alternative medicine internationally to support the claims of alternative practitioners, in comparison with the many such studies that have now become the touchstone of orthodox medicine (Ernst *et al.* 2001). Nonetheless, a growing number of small-scale trials have been conducted which suggest that certain alternative therapies may be more effective than placebos, and indeed than some mainstream orthodox remedies. Their effectiveness is well illustrated by a study of the employment of chiropractic for back problems, as against hospital outpatient care (see Meade *et al.* 1990). 'Scientific' medicine has also not always lived up to its own standards – given ethical and other difficulties in applying randomized controlled trials to many orthodox procedures (MacEoin 1990). To make matters even more problematic for the consumer in exercising an informed choice, methodological debates continue about whether such trials are the best method for evaluating more holistic alternative therapies. This is largely because such therapies are usually tailored to particular individuals, rather than being administered in a uniform manner for standard conditions (Lewith 1998). The need to control the placebo effect has also been countered because alternative practitioners often see this as a crucial element in its own right in the therapeutic armamentarium (Pietroni 1991).

What is clear, though, is that there are relatively high levels of consumer satisfaction with the outcomes of alternative therapy on both sides of the Atlantic (Sharma 1995; Astin 2000). This seems to be particularly true of chronic conditions, where orthodox medicine is at its most vulnerable. Although from a modernist perspective consumer satisfaction is problematic as an indicator of efficacy (Saks 1998a), it has certainly been a key driver in the rise of public interest in alternative medicine in Britain and the United States. However, not all aspects of the medical counter-culture have been so clear-cut as a driving force in relation to the rise of alternative medicine. This especially applies to the concept of 'holism', which has often been seen to lie at the heart of the various forms of unorthodox medicine that developed from the 1960s onwards (see, for example, Alster 1989). As Stalker and Glymore (1989) argue, a greater degree of scepticism may be called for here. Despite the centrality of this ideology, alternative medicine has not always or even perhaps mostly been holistic in practice, as was indicated at the outset of this volume. This is particularly so if the notion of 'holism' is broadly defined to include such features as the interdependence of mind, body and spirit; person-centred care; health as a positive state of being; open and reciprocal practitioner–client relationships; interprofessional involvement; and forging links between health and the wider social and physical environment (McKee 1988).

In this sense, it has become clear that not all practitioners of alternative medicine unite mind, body and spirit in their treatment (Peters 1998). For instance, Wardwell (1976: 65) has commented that osteopaths in the United States simply 'wanted to become fully-fledged medical practitioners and felt no incompatibility between the way they and the allopathic physicians conceptualize health, disease and therapy'. As this quotation suggests, and as will be seen in the next chapter, recent trends in the professionalization of alternative medicine also raise questions about the possibility of retaining a sense of equality in the relationship with the consumer in the Anglo-American context (Saks 2000b). Moreover, alternative therapists do not always work together with other health practitioners in a collaborative manner, using routinized referral networks for cases with which they are unable to deal. The lack of referral networks is exemplified by the individualistic practices of some exponents of unorthodox medicine in Britain, based on an entrepreneurial culture, that even inhibit the development of referral relationships between alternative practitioners themselves (Sharma 1995). In this vein, it is also rare for alternative practitioners to take into account wider socio-political factors, such as social class, in examining the client's position. Consequently, they can obscure rather than make transparent the political structures that lead to unhealthy environments and place unwarranted emphasis on individual solutions to health problems (McKee 1988).

Nevertheless, a number of alternative therapies have exhibited at least some dimensions of holism in Britain and the United States in recent years. Traditional Chinese acupuncturists, for instance, are concerned to balance the opposing forces of *yin* and *yang* that circulate through the meridians in linking mind, body and spirit. Classical homoeopaths also take a whole-person perspective in their efforts to influence the vital force by prescribing greatly diluted remedies to stimulate self-healing. Both types of therapy are further underpinned by the holistic principle of individualized diagnosis and treatment, taking into account emotional, physical and wider environmental influences (Fulder 1996). Holistic themes have also been manifested in the pioneering practice arrangements for alternative medicine that have increasingly sprung up in the Anglo-American context from the mid-1960s onwards. These range from the Bristol Cancer Help Centre and the Marylebone Health Centre in Britain (Pietroni 1991) to the network of Wholistic Health Centers on the East Coast and in the Midwest of the United States (Gordon 1981). Such settings focus on meeting the psychological and spiritual needs of the individual, while emphasizing self-help and the merits of a range of practitioners working collaboratively together. Some of the more holistic alternative practices, therefore, are potentially in conflict with the orthodox biomedical approach that aims directly to suppress or eliminate illness through the use of drugs, surgery and other mechanistic methods (Saks 1997a).

This challenge to the interests of orthodox biomedical practitioners from the revival of alternative medicine at a philosophical level was bolstered by the ensuing translation of public into political support for alternative medicine in Britain and the United States. This support provided a further threat to the power, status and financial position of organized medicine in both societies at élite and grassroots level. In Britain, as Saks (1992a) documents, such political support went over and above the lobbies of specific practitioner bodies in more popular areas such as acupuncture and homoeopathy – as well as representations from such umbrella organizations as the Institute for Complementary Medicine and the Council for Complementary and Alternative Medicine. It included the support provided by the still active all-Party Parliamentary Group for Alternative and Complementary Medicine, which was founded in the 1980s. Its work was enhanced by the active involvement of Prince Charles, who has wielded considerable influence in this field on behalf of alternative therapies – not least in his role of President of the British Medical Association and subsequently as the President of the Foundation for Integrated Medicine (Saks 1999c).

In the United States, too, political lobbies at federal and state level have complemented the work of specific individuals and organizations dedicated to advancing the cause of particular alternative therapies from herbalism to various forms of religious healing, in addition to the more generic holistic health movement (Alster 1989). Such support can be exemplified by the political impetus given to Traditional Chinese Medicine – and particularly Westernized forms of 'acupuncture anaesthesia' – as a result of the ping-pong diplomacy instigated by President Nixon in the early 1970s to open up diplomatic channels with China (Saks 1995b). This political impetus has been built upon by bodies such as the Coalition of Holistic Health Care Organizations, representing some 65 groups across the United States that came together in 1984 in Washington, DC (Heirich 1998). These and other lobbies paved the way for Congress to establish the Office of Alternative Medicine in 1992 – which has now grown into the National Center for Complementary and Alternative Medicine, designed proactively to promote research in this field (Cohen 1998). Such developments have added to the pressure on doctors on both sides of the Atlantic to put their own house in order through reform in the face of the medical counter-culture. How they have done so – and how their efforts have fitted in with their interests – is the subject to which the chapter finally turns.

THE MEDICAL RESPONSE TO ALTERNATIVE MEDICINE IN THE WAKE OF THE COUNTER-CULTURE

THE RESPONSE OF MEDICAL ORTHODOXY TO ALTERNATIVE MEDICINE IN BRITAIN

In Britain the leaders of the medical profession initially continued to be obstructive to reforms arising from the counter-culture. One example of this was the resistance of the General Medical Council in the 1970s to including all of the additional lay representatives recommended by the 1976 Merrison Committee on the regulation of the medical profession (Stacey 1992). Medical resistance to change, however, was especially apparent in the case of the response of the medical profession to alternative medicine. In the 1970s applications to become professions supplementary to medicine from both the osteopaths and chiropractors were turned down on medical advice (Fulder and Monro 1981). Even the existence of the handful of homoeopathic hospitals in the National Health Service that were the exception to the general rule in terms of state funding came under renewed challenge, as a result of action by local consultants (Inglis 1980). Leading medical journals such as the *British Medical Journal* and the *Lancet* also continued to report negatively on alternative therapies (see, for example, Saks 1991b). The ongoing adversarial climate between orthodox and alternative medicine was most apparent, though, in the report of the British Medical Association (1986) on alternative therapy. Much of the first half of the report was devoted to documenting the triumphant march of progress of orthodox biomedicine, in classic modernist fashion. In the remainder, alternative therapies were attacked for being 'unscientific', not least because of their link to medieval superstition and witchcraft.

This is not to say that the relationship between orthodox and unorthodox practitioners in this period was unchanged. The General Medical Council ended its ethical prohibition on referrals to alternative practitioners in the mid-1970s, with the proviso that doctors retained their control over treatment (Fulder and Monro 1981). While cooperation slowly grew, this did not immediately open up significantly greater collaboration with unorthodox medicine. Aside from the professional self-interests involved in an increasingly competitive area, doctors were inhibited by their legal obligations if they made referrals to non-medical practitioners in a relatively underdeveloped field. It also did not help that the British Medical Association continued to discourage such referrals in its advice to members, despite the shift in position of the General Medical Council (Fulder 1996), nor that the medically led 'quackbusting' Campaign Against Health Fraud – later to become Health-watch – launched a high-profile attack on alternative therapies from the late 1980s onwards (Walker 1994). Nonetheless, there was a growing trend for medical practitioners – especially in general practice – either to employ unorthodox medicine directly or to delegate such practice to health professionals within the orthodox division of labour, not least to nurses who were enthusiasts (Tovey 1997). Medical involvement in this field seems to have been fuelled in part by the legitimacy bestowed on it by gradually rising orthodox research investments into alternative medicine, as well as the appearance of more sympathetic items on this subject in the mainstream medical journals (Saks 1996).

In this light, a defensive stance towards medical unorthodoxy became less and less tenable, especially as pressure from the public and politicians increased in a pluralist political structure. Defensiveness threatened to lead, among other things, to the profession losing clients in the private sector in addition to some of its legitimacy. It was understandable, therefore, that a further, more sympathetic report was produced by the British Medical Association (1993) on what was now referred to as 'complementary medicine'. It argued that there should be greater collaboration between doctors and 'non-conventional' practitioners – with an appreciation of these therapies included in the medical school curriculum and more research undertaken into their effectiveness. The focus on unorthodox medicine shifted from outright dismissal, to defining how best alternative therapies could be regulated in future from the viewpoint of orthodox medical interests. Although the thrust of the report was apparently liberal, the interest-based interpretation of its contents is sustained by the support it gave to delegation to non-medical practitioners of alternative therapies under medical authority; its advocacy of a medically based core curriculum for unorthodox therapists, including subjects such as anatomy and physiology; and its continuing reliance on the biomedical touchstone of large-scale randomized controlled trials for evaluating unorthodox medicine (Saks 1996). This remains the policy of the medical profession, as endorsed by the latest report of the British Medical Association (2000) on acupuncture, one of the most popular of such therapies.

It should therefore not be surprising that certain alternative therapies are now directly employed by some 16 per cent of general practitioners and that access to these is provided by around 40 per cent of general practices, largely paid for by the National Health Service (Thomas *et al.* 1995). Most pain clinics also regularly use such therapies, which are typically administered by nurses and other orthodox health practitioners (Trevelyan and Booth 1994). This is increasingly underpinned by selective inputs on alternative medicine in undergraduate medical courses and other forms of higher and further education (see, for instance, Morgan *et al.* 1998). The benefit to the medical profession as a whole of incorporating such therapies in this way has been to counter the challenge from rival practitioners in the face of adverse public and political opinion, while minimizing the threat from outsiders. General practitioners, who historically have been at the sharpest end of market competition with unorthodox therapists, have particularly gained from their heightened engagement in the field. As Saks (1995b) indicates, their involvement has provided, among other things, increased opportunities for private practice in an area where this is relatively rare. They have also established further mechanisms for dealing with 'difficult' patients who are constantly returning with chronic conditions, about which orthodox medicine at present can do relatively little.

These factors help to explain in terms of interests why such therapies have generally been taken up with greater enthusiasm by generalists than by specialists in the acute sector – especially given the more directly controlled and elaborated career structure of the latter. In both the primary care and the acute sector, the manner in which alternative therapies have been incorporated into medical orthodoxy, without subverting its philosophical underpinnings, is also significant. A good example is acupuncture, which doctors have primarily employed as an analgesic on the basis of orthodox neurophysiological explanations of its *modus operandi* – including most recently those focused on endorphins (Saks 1992b). In contrast, the wide-ranging use of this therapy by many non-medical practitioners tends to be based on traditional Eastern philosophies that conflict with Western biomedicine. By responding to more challenging alternative therapies in this way, the medical profession has been able to restrict external threats to its income, status and power from an interest perspective. Adopting this strategy, it has also positively been able to create new fields to colonize in which its members, rather than its competitors, have ownership of the knowledge involved.

THE RESPONSE OF MEDICAL ORTHODOXY TO ALTERNATIVE MEDICINE IN THE UNITED STATES

In the United States the position taken by organized medicine in relation to the medical counter-culture was similar to that in Britain. Its initial resistance to change was apparent from its response to pressure from the feminist movement – indicated by the fact that even by the mid-1980s only 25 to 30 per cent of medical practitioners were women (Stacey 1985). Most importantly in this context, the leaders of the profession were also less than positively disposed towards many types of alternative medicine, their attitude being in part linked to the perceived challenge to medical interests. This took a variety of forms, ranging from the revoking of the state licensing of physicians using such therapies to the appearance of negative items about unorthodox therapies in mainstream medical publications (Cohen 1998). In this latter respect, for example, an aggressive stance was maintained towards chiropractic, which continued to be seen as 'unscientific' up to the 1980s by the leaders of the American Medical Association (Wardwell 1988). There were also ongoing attacks on other therapies. In 1981, for instance, the Food and Drug Administration sought to classify homoeopathic drugs as prescription items, a stance that threatened to eliminate lay prescribing (Kaufman 1988). At a more generic level, the National Council Against Health Fraud – paralleling the British 'quackbusters' tradition – waged war against unorthodox medicine by, among other things, striving to use restrictive state laws to limit the activities of individual practitioners of alternative medicine (Cant and Sharma 1999).

However, positive changes in the relationship between orthodox and unorthodox medicine based on incorporation have also occurred in the United States, as in Britain. Ever more physicians have taken up alternative medicine – with around 36 per cent practising at least one such therapy, the most popular of which are relaxation techniques and approaches based on lifestyle and diet (Cohen 1998). One of the most important indicators of the changing climate within mainstream medicine has been the formation of exclusive bodies of orthodox practitioners with common interests in alternative therapies. This is illustrated by the foundation of the American Holistic Medical Association, which emerged in the wake of the medical counter-culture from the late 1970s onwards and is centred predominantly on primary care physicians (Cant and Sharma 1999). Similar bodies in specific fields in Britain include organizations such as the Medical Acupuncture Society and the Faculty of Homoeopathy, which are also based on a restricted medical membership (Saks 2000b). Despite such parallels, though, the pattern of medical absorption of alternative therapies generally appears to have gone further and faster in the United States – notwithstanding variations in approach on an individual state-by-state basis in the more devolved American political system.

This pattern is very apparent in the case of acupuncture, which was more extensively and rapidly adopted by physicians in the United States than in Britain from the 1970s onwards – albeit with a predominant focus on pain and underpinned by orthodox neurophysiological theories in line with professional interests (Saks 1995b). That the level of the absorption of alternative medicine has generally been more advanced in the American context is also highlighted by the case of osteopathy, the practitioners of which have been incorporated into the medical profession itself in recent years. Their incorporation has involved the licensing of osteopaths as professional equals in every state (Wardwell 1994a). The price paid by the osteopaths, though, was a commitment to biomedically oriented training and practice. This has played a key part in diffusing the challenge that they might otherwise have posed to the interests of the medical profession had osteopathy been employed independently as a therapy for a broad band of conditions, with a competing philosophical base (Gevitz 1988a). This difference from Britain in the extent and speed of the medical incorporation of alternative therapies had already started to appear before the emergence of the counter-culture. Even by the 1960s, for instance, osteopaths had received orthodox acceptance in several American states, based on the growing convergence of the osteopathic curriculum with that of orthodox medicine (Baer 1987).

As in earlier times, the greater propensity for the American medical profession to adopt an incorporationist strategy again seems to have been related to the differential threat to its interests posed by medical outsiders within existing professional regulatory arrangements. In this respect, American physicians were unfettered by the common law rights that generally allowed the lay practice of alternative therapies in Britain. For that reason, physicians with control over licensing boards could have greater confidence about incorporating alternative therapies either by amalgamation, as in the case of the osteopaths, or by absorption, as with acupuncture. In the latter instance, from the 1970s onwards acupuncture was defined in most American states as a medical modality and licensed only for physicians or for those practising under the authority of a physician (Saks 1995b). The more restrictive licensing arrangements in the United States meant that physicians were able to respond positively to business opportunities related to public demand for alternative practice in a predominantly fee-for-service system without similar fears that doing so would legitimate rival bodies outside the profession.

This interest-based explanation of the different emphasis in the strategies employed by the American and British medical professions in response to alternative therapies in a competitive marketplace does not mean that incorporation has always been a comfortable process for medical orthodoxy in the United States. Indeed, the recently enhanced standing gained by chiropractors in relation to medical orthodoxy has been profoundly uncomfortable in terms of the interests of organized medicine in protecting its income, status and power. This change was largely forced upon the American Medical Association by a court ruling in the late 1980s that required it to end its boycott of chiropractors as this contravened the anti-trust laws (Wardwell 1994a). The effect was to give chiropractors a range of medical rights that proved unpalatable as far as orthodox medicine was concerned, as many chiropractors subscribed to a philosophical base that was more challenging to biomedicine than that of the osteopaths. In addition, the services of the more eclectic chiropractors were very popular – and offered a potential threat to the typically less well-rewarded generalists in the medical profession. This in part explains why practitioners of chiropractic relied on public support to advance their position through the legislature, rather than directly seeking medical patronage (Coburn and Biggs 1986).

The overall effect nonetheless has been for physicians and other orthodox health personnel in the United States to capitalize increasingly on the burgeoning market in alternative medicine from an interest perspective. In this regard, it has been estimated that out-of-pocket expenditure on alternative medicine in 1997 was $27 billion, which was comparable to the projected out-of-pocket expenditure for all American physician services in that year (Eisenberg *et al.* 1998). It is not surprising, therefore, that despite the traditional opposition of the American Medical Association, courses in alternative medicine are now offered at many medical schools and the enthusiasm of doctors for directly practising such therapies is fast expanding (Pavek 1995). A crucial watershed in this field was the publication of a special report to the National Institutes of Health entitled *Alternative Medicine: Expanding Medical Horizons* (1994), which contained the work of over two hundred contributors on research into unorthodox practices. This was followed in November 1998 by a positive themed issue of the *Journal of the American Medical Association* devoted to alternative therapies. These developments demonstrate that although there have been differences in the level of responsiveness, orthodox medicine in both Britain and the United States has not stood still in the face of the challenge of alternative medicine.

In this vein, the danger of overly stereotyping positions in analysing the relationship between orthodox and unorthodox medicine is underlined. This danger can be highlighted with reference to the concept of 'holism'. As was mentioned earlier in this chapter, this notion is not as fully applicable to the range of alternative therapies as their proponents would sometimes have us believe. On the other hand, orthodox biomedicine in the Anglo-American context has perhaps been portrayed as being more reductionist than it is, without acknowledging the changes that have been effected following the emergence of a strong counter-culture from the mid-1960s. These changes are accentuated by the current moves to incorporate alternative medicine into medical orthodoxy. There is also a realization in orthodox medical circles of the need for greater emphasis on enhancing the patient–practitioner relationship, as well as on the patient as an individual. In this respect, recent attempts have been made to improve the communication skills of doctors and other health professionals and to sensitize them to the social networks in which their patients are embedded (see, for example, Gordon 1988). Counsellors and social workers too have been increasingly involved in the delivery of orthodox medicine, as a growing appreciation has developed of the importance of self-care and the links between mind and body (see, for instance, Leathard 1994). Moreover, at a wider level there has been rising medical awareness of the impact of the socio-economic environment on health, as exemplified by developments in public health (Ashton and Seymour 1990; Weiss 1997).

Even so, there are definite limits on how far orthodox medicine has been holistically reformed in Britain and the United States. These are well illustrated by the bounded terms of acceptance of alternative therapies such as acupuncture within medical orthodoxy in the current climate. It is notable that the biopsychosocial model of Engel (1980), which has conceptually underpinned most efforts by doctors to transcend biomedical reductionism, is still based on a positivist medical tradition linked to the notion of the cell (Lyng 1990). Effective interprofessional cooperation with other health and social care workers has also all too often been restricted by relationships of medical dominance (as illustrated by Owens *et al.* 1995). Self-help has tended as well to become an appendage to orthodox medicine rather than a more radical alternative, with the concept of reciprocal client–practitioner partnerships subverted by the objectification of the patient within the modernist paradigm (Saks 1998a). In addition, there have been restrictions on how far public health initiatives are promoted in practice (Navarro 1994; Baggott 2000). Nonetheless, the adaptability of orthodox medicine has proved to be a crucial weapon in the interest-based politics of health care on both sides of the Atlantic, which has been regularly deployed in a rapidly changing health policy context in recent years. This shifting contemporary context and its implications for the medical profession in the two societies concerned are discussed in the next chapter, along with the growing trend towards the professionalization of alternative medicine.

NOTE

1. For simplicity, the references to Britain from the mid-twentieth century onwards focus on England and Wales, as there are some key differences in the system that developed in Scotland and Northern Ireland (see Levitt *et al.* 1995).

CHAPTER 5

Health policy, professionalization and the state

As we have seen from previous chapters, the nature and form of orthodox and alternative medicine have changed substantially in both Britain and the United States over the years. So too has the interrelationship between them. This chapter looks at one of the most significant current changes to unorthodox medicine in the interface with medical orthodoxy – namely, the way in which alternative practitioners have increasingly sought to professionalize. Their attempts to do so are ironic because, as we have seen, the marginalization of alternative therapies itself derived from the state-underwritten professionalization of medicine in an earlier era. However, before discussing this latest development, the chapter examines the major shifts in state health policy related to mainstream medicine from the early 1970s onwards in the Anglo-American context. Some of these changes can be seen as a response to the counter-culture of the 1960s and 1970s considered in the previous chapter. Still others reflect the growing economic pressures on the health care system in both societies over the past two or three decades. Whatever their causes, they have stimulated a key debate about their impact on the position of the medical profession on both sides of the Atlantic – and in particular about whether medicine has been deprofessionalized. The main theories about deprofessionalization are analysed in this chapter, as a prelude finally to discussing the recent intriguing trend towards the professionalization of alternative medicine.

SHIFTS IN STATE HEALTH POLICY IN BRITAIN AND THE UNITED STATES FROM THE 1970s

Technological changes in orthodox medicine in Britain and the United States continued to occur from the 1970s onwards (see, among others, Duin and Sutcliffe 1992; Le Fanu 1999). The development of computerized tomography (CT) and magnetic resonance imaging (MRI) scanners, for example, has enabled more and more parts of the body to be examined in detail from a diagnostic viewpoint. While 'smart' drugs have been introduced for an even wider range of conditions, surgeons have also increasingly employed powerful operating microscopes in micro-surgery in areas such as ophthalmology, neurosurgery and plastic surgery. The technology has become available too to produce 'test-tube babies' conceived by *in vitro* fertilization. At the same time, advances in genetic engineering and gene therapy have raised hopes for further health enhancement in the future. While the significance of these technological changes should not be understated, the public reception of such developments has been more restrained than in the heady days following the mid-twentieth century, after the counter-cultural backlash in the period from the mid-1960s to the mid-1970s (Saks 2000a). The influence of this period on orthodox medicine is also apparent to some extent in the organization of health care in Britain and the United States from the 1970s, an outline of the policies underpinning which is set out below.

HEALTH POLICY IN BRITAIN

In Britain the 1970s was a time when the National Health Service became still further consolidated, albeit not without significant reform. While the principle of a comprehensive state service free at the point of access was retained, the *Report of the Royal Commission on the National Health Service* (1979) suggested that further change lay ahead. The report was critical of the 1974 reorganization. This had established a more unified and coordinated service. However, it was argued, among other things, that decisions were still too often imposed from above and that there was a need for greater local integration between agencies. The incoming Conservative government of 1979 responded through the 1982 reorganization of the National Health Service by eliminating Area Health Authorities, leaving regions and districts as the key decision-making entities (Levitt *et al.* 1995). It also attempted to transcend the previous philosophy of consensus management, which often led to inertia, by following through the recommendations of the Griffiths Report (Department of Health and Social Security 1983). This supported the introduction of general managers at unit, district and regional levels, a move aimed at enhancing the efficiency and effectiveness of decision-making at a time when financial pressures on the National Health Service were growing. These were amplified by the development of new medical technologies, which, along with resource restrictions, added to the dilemmas of rationing and prioritization (Allsop 1995a).

The new Conservative government was very much wedded to the market. The Griffiths Report, which aimed to extend the principles of private-sector management into the National Health Service (Cox 1991), highlighted this. Attachment to market forces was also reflected in its encouragement to patients to make more use of private medicine, following the American model, as well as in its promotion of contracting out of the National Health Service for such services as laundry and catering (see, for instance, Higgins 1988). The market emphasis – which led to a tangible increase in business for the private sector (Allsop 1995a) – was strongly manifested too in the White Paper *Working for Patients* (Department of Health 1989). This sought to respond to rising public expectations, an ageing population, further advances in medical technologies, and the budgetary difficulties of the National Health Service. Even though health care remained primarily state funded, it paved the way for the introduction of an internal market into the National Health Service, centred on purchasers and providers. Market relations were to be based on the creation of hospital and community Trusts with their own management boards that would operate alongside general practitioner fundholders with their own patient-related budgets (Levitt *et al*. 1995). This White Paper complemented a number of other government policy initiatives, including *The Health of the Nation* (Department of Health 1992), which set out national targets in five major areas where mortality and morbidity rates could be reduced: coronary heart disease, cancers, mental illness, HIV/AIDS and sexual health, and accidents.

Such government health policies, however, were largely superseded in 1997 when the Labour administration came to power. The White Paper *The New NHS: Modern, Dependable* (Department of Health 1997) affirmed the commitment of the government to the National Health Service, while highlighting the departure from both the internal market and the previous centralized command structure. The motif for the modernized health system was to be partnership – aimed at overcoming market fragmentation, breaking down barriers between service agencies and professional groups, and fostering interdependence. Alongside this, a system of clinical governance was introduced in the health Trusts and the newly formed Primary Care Groups, the latter of which had commissioning powers. This was complemented by the introduction of an explicit information technology strategy and Health Action Zones, which aimed to address health inequalities through local partnerships (Department of Health 1998). A system of priorities was also affirmed in relation to cancer, coronary heart disease and stroke, accidents and mental illness (Department of Health 1999). At the same time, the new National Institute for Clinical Excellence and the Commission for Health Improvement took the lead on clinical and cost-effectiveness issues and the quality of clinical services respectively in an era of evidence-based medicine. Local strategic health developments, moreover, were to be centred on health improvement programmes coordinated by health authorities (Department of Health 1997).

This vision was developed in *The NHS Plan* (Department of Health 2000c). It outlines the commitment of government to, among other things, investment to reduce waiting times, enhanced information technology systems, extra hospital beds and improved premises in general practice. It also aims to establish a concordat with private providers to help the National Health Service make better use of private hospitals. This aim is associated with a desire to improve a range of services – from cancer screening to nursing care for the elderly – while reducing inequalities, not least by increasing the links between health and social care. The latest organizational changes designed to support the modernization of the health service are set out in a consultation document entitled *Shifting the Balance of Power within the NHS* (Department of Health 2001e). These include the abolition of Regional Offices of the Department of Health; putting in place Regional Directors of Health and Social Care; developing Primary Care Trusts as lead bodies; and establishing a smaller number of Strategic Health Authorities. The onus here is on empowering local communities and front-line staff, with appropriate central support. While the ability of the government to deliver its vision in this way remains to be demonstrated, the framework established certainly underlines the current intent to implement even greater change in health policy.

In this changing context, orthodox health professions in Britain have come under increasing challenge. This is illustrated by the implementation of systematic medical audit as a result of the reforms under the Conservative government (Levitt *et al.* 1995). The challenge to medical orthodoxy was evident too from the desire by the Thatcher government to subject professional groups to the rigours of the market, after it had taken on local authorities and trade unions. The attack on the restrictive powers of the health professions was primarily focused on the establishment of contractual relationships between purchasers and providers (Alaszewski 1995). The agenda of reforming the health professions was also taken forward under the new Labour government in its search for more flexible approaches to health care in the public interest, in the face of the increasing need for cost containment. The implementation of reform has been accelerated by rising political concern about the abuse of self-regulatory powers, particularly in medicine (see, for instance, Allsop and Mulcahy 1996). Recent issues have included the failure of the medical profession to pick up the deviant activities of the now convicted serial killer Dr Harold Shipman; the removal of organs by doctors without consent at the Alder Hey Children's Hospital in Liverpool; and the carrying out of surgery on children with unacceptably high mortality rates at the Bristol Royal Infirmary. These and other cases have led to efforts to curb the autonomous professional powers of doctors and cognate professional groups (Davies 1999).

Against this, the position of medicine – and the allied health professions – has continued to be strengthened by technological developments. These developments are highlighted by the expanding range of hospital specialisms, such that by the 1980s there were 54 categories of hospital medical staff in Britain (Larkin 2000). That said, a greater proportion of government expenditure than hitherto has been spent on primary care based on group practice in health centres, backed up by increasingly advanced medical equipment and information technology (Allsop 1995a). Nonetheless, such primary care amounts to only a quarter of National Health Service spending, although there is a relatively even split between the numbers of hospital specialists and general practitioners (Busfield 2000). Moreover, medical education since the 1970s has tended to remain hospital focused, notwithstanding recent reforms (Harrison *et al.* 1990). Despite funding shifts, hospital specialists still also attract the bulk of research resources from national funding bodies such as the Medical Research Council and the Department of Health (see, for example, Department of Health 2000b). However, primary care based on multi-professional teams containing self-employed general practitioners and a range of other workers in health and social care is now far more prevalent, with a growing policy emphasis on prevention and care in the community (Levitt *et al.* 1995). The form of health care provision is therefore discernibly changing as compared with the mid-1970s (Jones 1994).

Specialisms have also become more established in orthodox health professional fields such as nursing (Davies and Beach 2000). Here changes in technology, together with shifts in philosophy, have enabled the large, predominantly female nursing profession to take on more of the activities of doctors and delegate other tasks to health support workers – gaining power and status in the process. This trend has been accentuated by government policy (Alaszewski 1995), including the introduction of more robust educational provision for nurses under the auspices of Project 2000 from the late 1980s onwards (Witz 1994) and the implementation of parallel improvements in other professions allied to medicine (Levitt *et al.* 1995). *The NHS Plan* (Department of Health 2000c) has underlined the need for more and better-paid health staff with flexible working practices. In this context, the division of labour has been extended through the introduction of such roles as nurse and therapist consultants, while enhanced managerial and clinical leadership programmes are increasingly being provided for health professionals – along with financial assistance for the development of health support workers. The aim is to make the most responsive and effective use of staff, backed up by integrated workforce planning, tailored multidisciplinary training and education, and more flexible career structures. This strategy is more fully articulated in the consultation document *A Health Service of All the Talents: Developing the NHS Workforce* (Department of Health 2000a), in which the benefits of team-working across occupational and organizational boundaries are extolled.

Thus there is a need to be aware of linkages across, as well as divisions within, professions – in addition to the position of specific professional groups. The internal dynamics of professions are currently well exemplified by the changing balance of power between hospital specialists and general practitioners. The health reforms over the last two or three decades of the twentieth century have meant that the pendulum of dominance has begun to swing from hospital specialists more in the direction of general practitioners. The change has come about mainly because of the growing priority placed by the government on primary care and the increasing commissioning role given to general practitioners in the new National Health Service (Allsop 1995b). It is also important to underline the ever-wider range of allied orthodox health professional groups that make up the division of labour. These include not only nursing, but also the diverse span of subordinated and limited professions from physiotherapists and occupational therapists to pharmacists and dentists (Turner 1995). In all cases, change is in process in the new policy climate (Walby and Greenwell 1994), as is illustrated by the development of delegated roles like aides and assistants associated with such health professions and the growth of interprofessional education and practice in health and social care. This has not always been a smooth process, in part because the professional groups involved have typically sought to protect their own boundaries in line with their own interests (Davies *et al.* 2000).

The most important structural development in this context has been the government-inspired reviews of a number of health professions. Under the Conservatives, these led to the deregulation of optical services in 1984. The subsequent opening up of the sale of spectacles meant that the interest-based professional monopoly of opticians on dispensing was undermined (Saks 1987). More recently, formal reviews have been undertaken of nurses, midwives and health visitors (JM Consulting 1998) and the professions supplementary to medicine (JM Consulting 1996). As a result, the Nursing and Midwifery Council and the Council for Health Professions have been established in place of the United Kingdom Central Council and the English National Board for Nursing, Midwifery and Health Visiting, and the Council for the Professions Supplementary to Medicine respectively. The former change should lead, among other things, to a more streamlined register as a basis for the regulation of nursing and midwifery (Department of Health 2001a). The latter development is intended to enhance public confidence by establishing a smaller, more strategic council with a limited number of statutory committees, capable of responding more swiftly to change in the allied health field (Department of Health 2001d). The government has also proposed that the individual regulatory bodies be accountable to Parliament through a new overarching Council for the Regulation of Healthcare Professions (Department of Health 2001c).

Part of the impetus for changes to professional regulation has come from the desire for a more patient-oriented service. The greater focus on the public is perhaps the most significant legacy for orthodox medicine of the strong counter-culture that emerged in the late 1960s and early 1970s. This trend began in Britain in 1974 with the previously documented introduction of Community Health Councils. It was reinforced by the production of the consultative document *Patients First* (Department of Health and Social Security 1979), which emphasized the need for management of the National Health Service by local people. It advocated increasing representation of local interests on health authorities and greater flexibility for local managers in managing the health service (Allsop 1995a). It was followed under the Conservative government by the introduction of *The Patient's Charter* (Department of Health 1991), which explicitly set out the rights of patients and the standard of service that professionals were expected to provide. These rights ranged from receiving clear explanations of treatment and having access to clinical records to being provided with a named nurse. Thus it complemented the National Charter Standards introduced by the Department of Health and the more generic *Citizen's Charter* (Alaszewski 1995). It also paralleled the development of a more user-friendly and wider complaints system following the implementation of the 1990 Wilson Report (Levitt *et al.* 1995).

This stress on the importance of the increased involvement of the public in health care has been carried on – and possibly accelerated – in the policies of Tony Blair's Labour government. The Health Action Zone initiative is centred on local communities taking a lead in health reform (Department of Health 1998). The consumer has also now become central to some areas of the National Health Service previously considered taboo, such as research and development. As *The NHS Plan* (Department of Health 2000c: 88) makes clear, 'NHS care has to be shaped around the convenience and concerns of patients. To bring this about, patients must have more say in their own treatment and more influence over the way the NHS works.' The operationalization of this policy, though, has controversially signalled the end of Community Health Councils. However, patient-centred services are to be enhanced by the establishment of new Patient Advocacy and Liaison Services in the Trusts, dealing with the immediate concerns of patients and carers. It is also anticipated that Patients' Forums, with powers to inspect any aspect of the care process, will provide further leverage in effecting positive change in these settings (Department of Health 2001e).

This consumer-focused approach has added impetus to the reform of the orthodox health professions. This has gone furthest in the formation of the General Social Care Council – covering social work and related areas – on which the public and employers outnumber practitioners (Davies 1999). There is also greater lay membership on the new Nursing and Midwifery Council (Department of Health 2001a) and the Council for Health Professions (Department of Health 2001d). Indeed, even the General Medical Council has now increased its lay constituency – alongside the introduction of further reforms to enhance public confidence, including a scheme to regularly revalidate practising doctors (General Medical Council 2000). Such public representation in the health field is considered vital if the consumer is to be more fully protected and the quality of health care further improved. It is also crucial if persisting health inequalities are to be addressed. Although some more blatant geographical inequalities had been reduced (Allsop 1995a), significant issues remained for disadvantaged groups such as the lower social classes, women and certain ethnic minority groups (see, for example, Townsend and Davidson 1982; Whitehead 1987). Despite government denials, inequalities seem to have grown rather than diminished while the Conservatives were in power (Baggott 2000). The outcome of the inquiry by Acheson (1998), morever, underlined that there is still much work to be done in combating health inequalities under the Labour administration.

HEALTH POLICY IN THE UNITED STATES

Similar trends to Britain in relation to orthodox health care are evident in the United States, not least in terms of the political imperative to obtain value-for-money services within budgetary constraints over the past two or three decades. However, the structures of the two health systems remain substantially different. While federal, state and local government spending at various levels has now risen to make up over 40 per cent of total health expenditure in the United States (Chandler 1996), the American system has continued to be centred on private funding, mirroring the wider political framework. Inevitably, in a privatized system based mainly on individual fee payment and health insurance with limited central direction, additional costs have resulted from the lack of overall coordination. In this sense, it may be no coincidence that over twice the proportion of gross domestic product is currently invested in the health sector in the United States as compared to Britain (Moran 1999).

However, within the political parameters operating in the United States, cost containment became the major health issue from the mid-1970s onwards

(Starr 1982). This is not surprising, as costs have risen as a result of such factors as the development of medical technologies, which have been taken to a high point of refinement in the United States (McGuire and Anderson 1999). The traditional fee-for-service model on which the health system was based also gave too much of an incentive for providers to increase care beyond what was strictly necessary (Krause 1996). In addition, there were too few effective levers by the mid-1970s to keep costs in check in a predominantly market-oriented health system (Chandler 1996). The initial financial upshot was for stricter government limits to be introduced on health care payments. In the early 1980s the federal government froze physicians' fees for Medicare. The states also followed this example for Medicaid (Anderson 1989). The main longer-term vehicle for cost control was the establishment in 1983 of fixed prices for treatments according to federally determined Diagnostic Related Groups – each of which henceforth attracted a specified standard payment, regardless of the actual costs incurred (Higgins 1988). This system of cost control has had implications for the large number of for-profit hospitals and private nursing homes operating alongside non-profit hospitals, teaching hospitals and public hospitals in the American health system. They have had to hold costs down, albeit often at the risk of comebacks from releasing patients 'quicker but sicker' (Weiss 1997).

Managed care has also come more fully into the equation as a method of cost containment, with more than 135 million American enrollees in such plans at the beginning of the 1990s (Kalisch and Kalisch 1995). It differs from traditional American indemnity fee-for-service schemes by being based on features such as risk-sharing between insurers and providers, limitations on providers' autonomy, restrictions on patient choice and a degree of vertical integration of services. Many different forms of managed care are available, from Primary Care Case Management and Point of Service Plans to Social Health Maintenance Organizations. One of the fastest growing is that based on Preferred Provider Organizations. These offer lower premiums to subscribers as they negotiate fee-for-service discounts with particular doctors and hospitals in exchange for guaranteeing a certain volume of work within tightly controlled patterns of utilization. As such, they provide more choice than the wide range of different models of Health Maintenance Organizations that have significantly influenced their development (Robinson and Steiner 1998). Health Maintenance Organizations nonetheless have come to typify managed care and have proved increasingly significant since the 1970s. By the beginning of the 1990s there were some 550 in existence, with over 40 million subscribers (Weiss 1997).

Health Maintenance Organizations were initially pump-primed through federal funding in the Nixon era. Based on earlier pioneering initiatives like the Kaiser-Permanente scheme, they are centred on offering comprehensive group and basic hospital services on a pre-paid fee basis (Chandler 1996). In this respect, they are intended to provide a mutual interest incentive for both salaried doctors and patients to restrict the size of bills by focusing on early diagnosis, prevention and outpatient treatment – thereby reducing the demand for hospital care (Higgins 1988). The drive to limit costs is also reflected in their growing absorption into larger corporate networks, which contrasts with their roots as consumer-run, cooperative organizations (Starr 1982). In this sense, the introduction of managed care through Health Maintenance Organizations and other schemes, alongside Diagnostic Related Groups, has been associated with the increasing corporatization of medicine in the United States. This has been expressed in the growing concentration of fewer, larger organizations in this field and an expanding proportion of for-profit chains owning acute beds and managing hospitals themselves. A similar clustering of not-for-profit hospitals has also occurred. This helps them to respond to financial pressures, highlighted by the initial decrease in profitability of the companies involved in the private sector (Higgins 1988).

With some 70 per cent of Americans now in managed care plans (Marmor 1998), though, Health Maintenance Organizations and managed care in general have come under serious challenge. The efficiency of such schemes has been disputed for a variety of reasons, including the fact that they do not in practice reduce health care expenditure because they enlarge administrative costs for insurers and providers (Sullivan 2001). The priority given to preventive health too has not been as great as anticipated, as American medicine has increasingly been drawn into the world of large-scale corporate business in the for-profit sector (Chandler 1996). This business environment has led the companies concerned to move into new areas such as adolescent psychiatry and chemical dependency, on the basis of profitability fuelled by demand (Higgins 1988). While this move has had some positive effects, there has been a consumer backlash centred on the belief that managed care compromises the quality of health provision (Hellander 2001). The backlash has prompted some of the plans to allow more ready access to a wider range of specialists, partly as a result of the fear of litigation (Baucher 2001). On the other hand, providers are worried about reductions in hospital profitability and relatively low levels of physician reimbursement, as the income of managed care organizations falls (Sekhri 2000). It is not surprising in this light that a substantial number of Health Maintenance Organizations went bankrupt and/or were merged or acquired during the 1980s and 1990s (Weiss 1997).

At the same time, employers – now the largest subscribers to health insurance plans – have sought to restrict their liability in face of rising costs. They have done so in part by limiting the services to which their employees are entitled, including by requiring a contribution from them (Higgins 1988). This in turn has impacted on a health care system that, as we saw in Chapter 4, is already pervaded by deep-seated inequalities. Kalisch and Kalisch (1995) note that approximately 17 per cent of Americans have been adjudged to have inadequate access to physicians – with the absence of health insurance coverage being the biggest obstacle, especially for the poor. At the same time, impoverished inner-city populations with large black populations have mortality rates that are twice those of their fellow Americans. Some progress has been made in addressing such inequalities. One example is the establishment in the 1980s of the Office of Minority Health by the United States Department of Health and Human Services (1985). This has been active as a focal point for reducing disparities in black health, as access to health has improved for black Americans (Rice and Winn 1991). Another illustration is the increase in the supply of graduate physicians in deprived rural areas in the late 1980s and early 1990s (Krause 1996). However, there are still large socio-economic inequalities in health, and Moss (2000) believes these need to be given greater priority through multi-sectoral alliances, state and community task forces, and other mechanisms.

One of the biggest priorities for the United States, however, is addressing the persisting lack of health insurance cover for disadvantaged groups. It is estimated that the number of Americans without medical insurance has now risen to 45 million, comprising one in every six citizens (Baucher 2001). Shi (2001) points out that although low income is the most significant predictor of lack of insurance coverage, some ethnic minorities are over-represented in this group. This issue has been much debated in political circles in the United States. As Chandler (1996) observes, it has been argued for several decades that there is a need to base the United States health care system on the principle of universal coverage, as in Britain and many other European states. Forward movement was restricted under President Carter in the latter part of the 1970s because of the priority given to limiting the dramatically rising costs of health care, despite his election pledge to introduce comprehensive national health insurance. Thereafter, consideration was delayed by the election in 1980 of President Reagan, a Republican who stood on a pro-free market platform and reversed a number of redistributive policies during his two terms in office (Marmor 1998). President Bush fared little better, despite questioning as to why the United States did not have a national health plan providing universal and comprehensive health benefits to all its citizens (Navarro 1992).

However, President Clinton endeavoured to progress this agenda when he came to power on the Democratic ticket in 1992, in the wake of a remarkable consensus for reform that had built up in the United States and a commitment to restructure American health care (Marmor 1998). Proposals were announced in 1994 to establish a compulsory system of comprehensive health insurance, based on regional alliances administered by a national health board empowered to buy health services from hospitals and doctors. In this model, the states were to ensure that overall coverage was comprehensive, and individuals, families and employers were to make payments where appropriate. However, this scheme, centred on managed competition, did not take off. Many explanations have been given for the debacle, which even now may still require deeper political analysis (Hacker 2001). These range from the distractions of foreign policy, the end of the recession and the lengthy time taken in developing the scheme (Marmor 1998) to resistance from the Republican Party, supported by the American Medical Association and health insurance companies (Chandler 1996). Whatever the reasons, radical reform seems unlikely in the foreseeable future, as is underlined by the plans of the new President, George W. Bush Jr, which span from converting Medicare into a Health Maintenance Organization voucher programme to promoting medical savings accounts (Hellander 2001).

That said, there are many parallels with Britain as regards mainstream health policy. Strong efforts in the United States are being made to improve the quality of care. Key bodies here include the Institute of Health Improvement, together with the Joint Commission Accreditation of Healthcare Organizations, which reviews hospitals, and the National Council of Quality Assurance, which provides voluntary services for primary care elements of managed care companies (Botelho 2000). The current administration has made a commitment too to roll out information technology further into the health care workplace and to continue to support biomedical research in the United States – with a rising overall budget for the National Institutes of Health of at least $20 billion (Baucher 2001). Furthermore, paralleling the policy of successive British governments, the United States Department of Health and Human Services (2000) has released *Healthy People 2010*, which sets out its longer-term national health goals, aimed at enhancing life expectancy and the quality of life, as well as eliminating health disparities. Although the targets are more ambitious and cover a wider span of areas, from cancer and diabetes to oral health and physical activity, there are many similarities with Britain. This is also true of the reduction of the scale of the American hospital sector related to cost, technological developments, changing patient expectations and other factors (Kalisch and Kalisch 1995).

Differences in health policy between the two systems, though, continue to abound. These are well illustrated by the pivotal case of primary care. Whereas in the United States there has been a shift from hospitals towards ambulatory care, outpatient visits, home care and care in physicians' offices, the development of primary care has not been as extensive as in Britain.

Although it has come more to the fore with Health Maintenance Organizations and other types of managed care – given their cost-saving focus on promoting wellness in such areas as smoking cessation and counselling – there remain marked distinctions from Britain. Starfield (1997) notes that health care in the United States does not yet routinely encompass the main aspects of primary care, such as a common point of first contact for the patient, long-term person-focused care, a comprehensive range of services, and the coordination of provision. There have been attempts to place more policy emphasis on primary care. These are exemplified by the mandate given to Medicare by Congress in the mid-1980s to award higher fee increases in this area, and by government support for care in the community in mental health (Chandler 1996). However, primary care has generally been marginalized in the health reforms that have taken place to date (Starfield and Oliver 1999).

However, if primary care has not been a strong priority in America over the past two or three decades, this is perhaps to be expected in a country that still has a much lower proportion of generalist physicians than in Britain (Weiss 1997). The trends towards medical specialization have continued to be based on the development of new health care technologies, as is highlighted by rising subscriptions to the specialty associations of the American Medical Association, at a time when its overall membership is declining (Krause 1996). Chandler (1996) notes that it is in the interests of doctors in the United States to become specialists, as specialists usually command higher fees. The problem for consumers is that because of the lack of generalists, they are faced with not having a physician with an overarching understanding of their health and having to decide which specialist to visit – even if such practitioners will see patients in their own surgery and attend them in hospital. Although there is an increasing trend towards group practice by physicians (Starr 1982), the predominance of specialists in a strongly market-based system also means that orthodox health care is less joined up than in Britain at present, with a greater stress on competition than collaboration (Botelho 2000).

This competition is accentuated by the interest-based political manoeuvring that has taken place between physicians, the government and other health workers since the 1970s. Krause (1996) observes that the American Medical Association allowed the ratio of doctors to the population to double between 1970 and 1990 – to a position where previous restrictions on supply were loosened and there was an apparent oversupply of new physicians. This seems to have been brought about by the short-term interest of the profession in delivering the growth sought by government, in view of the dependence of medical schools on federal funding for research and the stipends that were given to them for each extra student trained. Nonetheless, the salaries of physicians could have been detrimentally affected in the longer term by this process in one of the most heavily doctored countries in the world (Starr 1982) – particularly in view of the cost-squeezing effects of the increasing number of independent private third-party plans and state regulatory programmes. It is testimony to the continuing strength of the profession that doctors' incomes actually grew by 30 per cent in the latter half of the 1980s to levels more than 50 per cent higher than those of their Canadian counterparts (Marmor 1998).

Nevertheless, the development of a profession that is becoming more salaried than self-employed in a corporate world in which its practitioners and other health professionals are increasingly responsible to well-paid business administrators has led Krause (1996) to question the continuing power of medical orthodoxy. For him, this is highlighted by the fact that the judgement of physicians is now more systematically subjected to professional review, fees are set on the basis of Diagnostic Related Groups, and greater lay control is being applied through managed care. In addition, this new context has increased divisions between specialist groups within the medical profession, including over which group should be best rewarded in terms of federal funding. Krause also notes that the American Medical Association no longer automatically has a place on the state licensing boards and national accrediting boards of other health professions. For instance, psychiatrists have lost authority over clinical psychologists, who can now practise in a number of states without medical supervision – as well as collect payments from Blue Cross. Pharmacists too are allowed to prescribe drugs independently in many states, while nurses routinely undertake admissions, diagnosis and treatment in less complicated cases in many for-profit hospitals to cut costs.

Even though physicians remain responsible for their own professional clinical training in accredited medical schools (Chandler 1996), therefore, there is little doubt that their position has changed since the 1970s. The fact that change has occurred is accentuated by recent cases of turf wars between medicine and other professional groups. The male-dominated profession of medicine has not always been successful in such battles, even in conflicts with predominantly female professional colleagues with a history of subordination to physicians (Hafner-Eaton 1994). Nurse practitioners, for example, have taken on the American Medical Association and local state medical associations with some success in their desire to become autonomous primary care providers (Kalisch and Kalisch 1995). Indeed, nursing – which, as in Britain, is by far the largest professional group – has been one of the more significant contemporary thorns in the side of medicine. Its emergence in that role can be traced back to the support that it received from the National Commission on Nursing in 1980 to be given more responsibility over decisions about patient care in hospital settings, including policy-making. As the level of qualifications of nurses in ever more specialist roles has risen, moreover, so tensions with physicians have grown – not least over such issues as the scope of the role of the certified nurse anaesthetist (Raffel and Raffel 1994).

Nurses were also the ultimate victors when the American Medical Association strove in the late 1980s to develop a new allied health profession, the registered care technologist, who, it was planned, would train and practise under the direct authority of physicians. This proposal was withdrawn after vigorous opposition from the American Nursing Association and more than a hundred other nursing organizations (Weiss 1997). Its defeat underlines the interest-based struggles that have occurred between non-medical health professions too. These include struggles between the professions subordinated to medicine and limited professions such as dentistry and pharmacy. There have also been demarcation disputes between physician assistants and members of other allied health occupations, of which 28 are accredited by the American Medical Association (Raffel and Raffel 1994). Registered nurses themselves have come under pressure from the non-professional and unlicensed nurses in the hospital sector who have displaced them – in some cases as a result of managerial strategies related to cost containment (Brannon 1996). In this regard, there have been tensions between health professionals as a whole and the increasingly graduate school-educated health administrators, whose importance has grown in the management of resources in corporate America (Krause 1996).

The outcome of such conflicts clearly impacts on the quality of care given to the consumer – whose role in developments in orthodox medicine over the past two to three decades has increased, as in Britain. In Chapter 4, the currently growing emphasis in the United States health care system on obtaining consumer rights was highlighted (Starr 1982). This has since been built upon with even more extensive public involvement in health care (Chandler 1996) – spanning from self-help and consumer lobbies for health action to representation on state licensing bodies and managed care plans. In the case of Health Maintenance Organizations, for instance, the federal government requires that a minimum of one-third of the board of directors are consumer members and that members of the local community are on boards covering under-served areas (Weiss 1997). In addition, Rodwin (1996) observes that the consumer voice in managed care has been amplified through individual complaint and grievance procedures. He also notes that there are four further strands to present policy approaches to consumer protection in health in the United States: product regulation, regulating marketing, promoting market competition, and ensuring the financial stability of firms involved in this area.

Most of these approaches depend on the law. In this respect, McGuire and

Anderson (1999) emphasize that patients have continued to follow the American tradition of relying on the law when their health care expectations are not met, by forming advocacy groups, hiring lawyers and seeking to initiate legislation. The courts have therefore remained crucial to public involvement in health care in the United States. A mandated change in the gender ratio of medical students based on anti-discrimination laws, for example, raised the proportion of females in medical school classes to at least a third by the early 1990s (Krause 1996). This rise helped to edge the gender balance closer towards the position in Britain, where women now constitute more than 50 per cent of medical students (Levitt *et al.* 1995). The law is a double-edged sword as far as the health professions are concerned. While it has underpinned many professional projects in this field, it has also been used against health professional groups. Patients in the United States now not only directly sue physicians for medical error, as in Britain (Baucher 2001), but also take litigation against the health plans under managed care for shortfalls in the quality of care (Sekhri 2000). The widespread use of litigation raises the question of whether these and other changes in the health terrain have led to the deprofessionalization of medicine in the contemporary Anglo-American context.

THE DEBATE OVER THE DEPROFESSIONALIZATION OF MEDICINE

The ground here has certainly shifted as compared with the period up to the mid-1960s when a strong counter-culture emerged. At that time, the professional standing of physicians in Britain and the United States was in little doubt. Medicine was widely regarded by social scientists as a classic profession, with one of the highest levels of income, status and power in society (Macdonald 1995). Neo-Weberian contributors variously held that the medical profession had significant levels of autonomy concerning the organization of its work (Freidson 1970) and was able to define the needs of the consumer and how these were to be satisfied (Johnson 1972). However, following the rise of the counter-culture, the literature from the 1970s onwards has been pervaded by claims about the 'deprofessionalization' of medicine, particularly in the United States (see, for instance, Haug 1973, 1988). This has also been depicted in Marxist accounts, which place more emphasis on the place of the medical profession in a capitalist economy, in terms of the related concepts of 'proletarianization' and 'corporatization' (see, for example, McKinlay and Arches 1985; McKinlay and Stoeckle 1988). The key question, however, is whether the changes in the position of the medical profession documented in this and the previous chapter indicate that it is on the wane on either side of the Atlantic. The focus here is on medicine, rather than other health professions, as this is the crucial litmus test of the strength of the orthodox health system given its long-standing dominance in the sector (Coburn 1999).

The critical macro-changes to which the deprofessionalization literature typically refers range from increasing state engagement, growing bureau-cratization and escalating corporate involvement in medicine to the developing challenge from other health professions and the rise of consumer power in health care. As Elston (1991) observes, these shifts are held to be leading, or to have led, to a variety of adverse effects from the viewpoint of the medical profession. At one end of the spectrum, they are seen to have diminished the degree of control by doctors over areas such as medical education and training, the terms on which work in medicine is carried out, and medical remuneration. At the other, they are held to have contributed to increasing encroachment by non-medical health personnel on the dominant position of doctors in the division of labour, the deskilling of medical work and growing public influence over medicine. In some Marxist accounts too, these trends are claimed to find expression in the growing unionization of physicians, as alienation is said to have increased. While acknowledging that changes have occurred in the health arena in both Britain and the United States, though, the deprofessionalization thesis remains open to debate – not least in charting the effects of wider shifts in the health care framework in which the medical profession operates.

In this regard, Stevens (1986) and Freidson (1994) recognize that the face of health care is changing, without accepting that the changes signal the end of medical ascendancy. The water is also muddied by ambiguities in the literature about the precise benchmarks being used in examining empirically how far the deprofessionalization of medicine has taken place and the timescales involved in the claims being made (Light 1995). In this latter respect, there are differences between its proponents over whether this process is in train or has already occurred, as well as the historic time line against which comparisons are to be made with the contemporary era. There are also disputes over the reasons why such changes are held to be occurring in the first place (Annandale 1998). As Elston (1991) observes, this confusion has meant that the deprofessionalization and other related theses have not as yet been satisfactorily developed in such a form that they are amenable to rigorous testing. It cannot be assumed either that any conclusions reached about the extent of the deprofessionalization of medicine in one society necessarily apply to another, not least because of international variations in the relationship between professions and the state (Larkin 1993). For this reason, the outline commentary that follows on the applicability of this type of theory in the Anglo-American context deals with Britain and the United States as separate entities, with the recognition that the outcome of any evaluation must be provisional.

THE APPLICABILITY OF THE DEPROFESSIONALIZATION THESIS TO BRITAIN

In Britain, as we have seen, a number of relevant trends have occurred. These include the move of doctors away from autonomous solo fee-for-service practice to work in larger bureaucratic settings, not least in the National Health Service. This move has meant that a greater proportion of the medical workforce – particularly in the hospital sector – is salaried and that doctors increasingly work within a more defined structure of management (Levitt *et al.* 1995). This is illustrated by the limited prescription list imposed on doctors in the late 1980s and the cash limits applied to general practitioners in the first half of the 1990s. It is clear too that doctors in Britain have not been totally their own masters in relation to either pay or medical education, where state financing restricts both levels of medical remuneration and curricula change (Elston 1991). At a more generic level, it is apparent that the medical–Ministry alliance is no longer as close as in the period before the emergence of a strong counter-culture. The weakening of the links is illustrated by the lack of consultation with the profession by the government over the introduction of the internal market into the health service in the late 1980s, a factor that played an important part in the vociferous protest of the British Medical Association against this (Crompton 1990).

Nonetheless, it is difficult to accept that medicine has as yet been deprofessionalized in Britain. One of the main reasons why this has been suggested is the state intervention that occurs through the National Health Service. In the United States, state intervention conjures up images of 'socialized medicine', which is associated with the demise of the autonomy of the medical profession. However, a salaried status coupled with state intervention is not necessarily incompatible with the existence of a range of autonomous powers. As Larkin (1993: 91) says, if state supervision emerges at an early historical stage – as opposed to being developed latterly in a 'free market' situation – 'it may actually but conditionally promote medical hegemony'. In Britain medical ascendance certainly appears to have risen in economic terms. Elston (1991) notes that although doctors in Britain have not been able to dictate their terms of service in the same way that is possible in a fee-for-service system, the manner in which they have organized themselves has given them considerable financial benefits. In this sense, the National Health Service has acted as a shelter from economic uncertainty for the medical profession, with a long-term alliance with the state providing its members with levels of pay well above those of most other occupational groups. Indeed, as she observes, a fee-for-service system does not guarantee a high income, as this depends, among other things, on there being sufficient demand for services from a paying clientele.

At the same time, the maintenance of significant clinical autonomy in medicine in the state-funded National Health Service has enabled the profession substantially to influence the use of government resources. The vehicles for such influence have ranged from representation on policy-making bodies at all levels to relative freedom from direct managerial supervision in practice (Klein 1989). As regards the latter, the general managers introduced with the Griffiths Report mainly served to draw more doctors into management roles, without abrogating their authority (Strong and Robinson 1990). Moreover, while the internal market provided stronger levers with which to influence clinical activity, it also helped to empower some groups of doctors – most notably general practitioners, who acted as purchasers of services on behalf of the public (Allsop 1995b). Even now, despite the determination of the Labour government to curb the medical profession in the face of growing evidence of the abuse of its powers, the principle of self-regulation, while tempered, has not been substantially subverted (Department of Health 2001c). The level of clinical autonomy of the British medical profession is therefore still quite great in the bureaucratized context of the National Health Service, even if external control over medical decision-making is beginning to increase. Such control is particularly apparent with the introduction of clinical governance, for which Trust chief executives are themselves responsible (Busfield 2000).

Change, then, does seem to have impacted on the position of the medical profession in Britain, but not to such a degree that it can now be said to be in disarray. The effect of change may well have been to reconstruct relationships between groups within medicine, rather than to subvert the profession as a whole. The process of restratification within the profession is best illustrated by the way in which general practitioners have improved their standing in relation to hospital specialists, as political priorities in health have shifted towards primary care (Allsop 1999). Moreover, change affecting the position of doctors does not seem to have markedly diminished their authority over other health professional groups – despite the enhanced position of nurses and associated personnel in the orthodox health care division of labour (Saks 1998b). Previously documented trends towards specialization, delegation and interprofessional working have had a limited impact in this area, largely because of the successful interest-based tactics of leaders of the medical profession in dealing with competitors. The skilful use of such tactics was highlighted in Chapter 4, in the way in which unorthodox practices have been incorporated into mainstream medicine over the past decade, in a manner designed to preserve the authority of the medical profession (Saks 1999b).

Yet if a high degree of professional control has been maintained in the rapidly changing British health care context, what of the challenge to doctors' professional standing by the public? As has been seen, since the mid-1970s in Britain a more patient-centred health service has been created, bolstered by government initiatives and direct consumer lobbies, following the development of the counter-culture (Elston 1991). The recently spiralling numbers of complaints against doctors indicate the extent of this challenge (Allsop and Mulcahy 1999). However, this challenge has not as yet significantly diminished the position of the medical profession. It has been variously countered by the inadequacy of the channels for the public to complain about clinical competence (Rosenthal 1987), the resilience of bodies such as the General Medical Council in responding to the views of the public (Stacey 1992), and the restricted powers of Community Health Councils (Fereday 1999). While increasing, health litigation is also currently less likely to be used by consumers in Britain as compared to the United States (Saks 2000a), although the distinctions can be overstated (Dingwall 1994). Members of the medical profession in Britain may be to a larger degree structurally insulated from the influence of the consumer too because of the greater salaried, as opposed to fee-for-service, context of their practice (Freidson 1970).

Opportunities for private medical practice are still far less extensive in Britain than in the United States, even if they are now expanding with the growth of large profit-oriented companies (Busfield 2000). This relative lack of opportunity, together with the comparatively weak market situation of many private hospitals in Britain (Elston 1991), indicates that the impact of corporatization has been much less significant here than on the other side of the Atlantic (Griffith *et al.* 1987). This is not to deny that the influence of corporate capitalist structures on health care in general and the medical profession in particular may be intensifying in Britain. A number of general commentaries on the political economy of health have indeed noted such a change (see, for example, Doyal 1979). This change has also been highlighted in more specific accounts about the influence of multinational corporations on medical consciousness through such mechanisms as conference and research funding by the pharmaceutical industry (Gould 1985). However, such arguments need to be treated with great care. The existence of the mainstream, state-funded National Health Service has limited the impact of corporate interests in Britain (see, for example, Higgins 1988). Moreover, the notion that their restricted, but increasing, influence has led to the deprofessionalization of medicine flies in the face of continuing evidence of the relative independence of the actions of doctors in Britain – as is pertinently illustrated in this context by the medical response to alternative medicine (Saks 1995b).

Nonetheless, in the face of change, the British medical profession has not completely retained the pre-eminent position that it held before the rise of the medical counter-culture, when the medical–Ministry alliance was at its peak (Saks 2000a). However, as Elston (1991) says, the challenges faced by orthodox medicine have not yet brought about its deprofessionalization in Britain. In addition to the points already discussed, growing trends towards specialization do not suggest that the medical profession has yet been de-skilled. Furthermore, doctors do not seem to have been sucked into widespread industrial action driven by alienation – notwithstanding the legal redefinition of their main representative body, the British Medical Association, as a trade union (Harrison *et al.* 1990). While the profession has undergone a substantial, and sometimes uncomfortable, readjustment in the cash-limited state health service, therefore, as Allsop (1999: 172) relates, it 'has accommodated to the changes and still maintains cultural, social and clinical autonomy over the content of its expertise'. The position in the United States can be interpreted a little differently – particularly, but not exclusively, because of the greater and ever-growing recent corporate influence over health care.

THE APPLICABILITY OF THE DEPROFESSIONALIZATION THESIS TO THE UNITED STATES

As we have seen, substantial changes in medicine have also occurred in the United States during the past two or three decades. As in Britain, there has been a general shift away from doctors working in single-handed practice settings to employment in larger organizations (Moran 1999), despite an increased tendency to move from hospitals back to office practice (Light 1993). While the pay levels of physicians remain relatively high (Marmor 1998), there has been the development of a salaried service – such that by 1990 more than half of doctors in the United States were on salaries (Krause 1996). As will be recalled, this change is linked to the emergence of bureaucratic management structures in which doctors are more accountable to business administrators, with the judgements of physicians increasingly being exposed to professional utilization reviews in wider organizational contexts (Moran and Wood 1993). Starr (1982) interprets this pattern as representing a decline in solo fee-for-service practice and the rise of corporate medicine. He emphasizes that the United States has moved a long way from nineteenth-century medical sovereignty, to a position where health care has become a largely corporate practice involving capitalism and the state. The key issue here, though, is whether this and other, parallel developments have had significant consequences for the standing of the medical profession – and, most importantly, whether they have led medicine down the road to deprofessionalization.

There are two main distinctions from Britain in relation to the above trends. The first is that the growth of the practice of working within large organizations has come later than in the British context, where there is a much stronger tradition of state intervention in health care (Larkin 1993). The second is that whereas both societies have capitalist economic structures, the growth of corporatization in the United States has been based more heavily on the expansion of the private sector (McKinlay and Stoeckle 1988). As we have seen, in this privatized framework the development of health insurance and managed care plans – in tandem with the increased power of multinational corporations (McKinlay 1984) – has brought with it huge financial pressures to limit costs. Largely as a result of these pressures, private third-party plans have since the 1970s increasingly become independent of the control of doctors (Krause 1996). This has, in turn, put pressure on the level of physician reimbursement, one of the key aspects of the deprofessionalization thesis. The clinical autonomy of physicians also seems to have been reduced, arguably as part of a process of proletarianization – which has meant closer scrutiny of mistakes and other aspects of their work situation (Starr 1982). McKinlay and Arches (1985) emphasize the role of managers in subordinating medical practitioners to the requirements of the corporations for which they work. This observation, however, needs to be balanced by the claim by Freidson (1994) that although professional workers may increasingly need to take orders, they typically take them from those who are already professionally qualified, or operate against criteria generated by professional peers.

The apparent decline of the profession is not just relevant to doctors working in the private corporations, which run some one-third of hospitals and the vast majority of home nursing (Krause 1996). It also applies to the public sector in the United States, which, unlike in Britain, appears not so much to have provided a shelter from the market as to have intensified the subordination of the medical profession within a corporate framework (McKinlay and Arches 1985). While physicians have found ways to turn the dependence of public and private corporations on their cooperation into authority and privilege (Derber *et al.* 1990), the growing federal, state and local government expenditure on health care has imposed significant constraints on them. These are best illustrated by the Diagnostic Related

Groups associated with Medicare, which were set up to provide common payments for given procedures based on reimbursable lengths of hospital stay. It is indicative of current trends that these payments were extended to include fee schedules for office visits from the late 1980s in order to reduce costs, by increasing health care in the community in place of more expensive specialist surgery (Krause 1996). This has clearly impinged on the autonomy of the medical profession. So too has the recent financial leverage employed by government to fund extra medical school places, which, as we have seen, has led to an expansion of the profession that has limited the long-term benefits of its restrictive monopolistic position (McKinlay and Stoeckle 1988).

In addition to such indicators of deprofessionalization, while doctors in the United States formally remain in control of their own professional training, they have come under serious challenge from other orthodox professional groups. As noted earlier, physician representation on state licensing boards and national accrediting boards of the allied health professions has declined over the past few years. The profession has also increasingly allowed the replacement of functions previously undertaken by physicians, such as drug prescribing, to be carried out by groups such as nurses and pharmacists, who can now operate independently in some states (Krause 1996). As documented previously too, doctors seem to have come off second best in a number of turf battles with other subordinated health professionals (see, among others, Kalisch and Kalisch 1995; Weiss 1997). In this sense, the interest-based tactics of the medical profession in the United States have not generally proved as successful as in Britain – even though the incorporation of some forms of alternative medicine has typically been advantageous to the profession (see, for example, Gevitz 1988a; Saks 1995b). Such trends have led McKinlay and Stoekle (1988: 192) to suggest that in America: 'Displaced by administrators, doctors have dipped down to the position of middle management where their prerogatives are also challenged or encroached upon by other health workers.'

Against this, the more intensive specialization of medicine in the United States, usually based on the development of ever more esoteric technological knowledge, has limited the extent to which it can be said to have been deskilled within the terms of the deprofessionalization thesis. At the same time, specialization is a potential danger to the medical profession. McKinlay and Stoekle (1988) see it as providing greater opportunity for the delegation of tasks to other health personnel, especially with the growing ideology of non-hierarchical team working. But if such delegation hints at a possible loss of control, the increasing divisions to which growing specialization has given rise may also have weakened the profession (Krause 1996). This is nowhere more apparent than in the previously documented current battle between medical specialists over the level of federal funding that each group should receive.

Although there has not been a realignment of the relative positions of specialists and generalists as in Britain, Freidson (1989) argues that some restratification has occurred in the new order between the rank and file and the élite, centred on the division of managerial functions within the profession. Where he and some other commentators part company is on how far the clinical autonomy of medicine has been significantly affected by such trends.

Another argument that medical autonomy has been substantially eroded in the United States is centred on the increasing challenge from the public, prompted by the emerging counter-culture. Haug (1973) bases her claims about deprofessionalization on the changing relationship between professionals and consumers – and, in particular, on the decreasing knowledge gap between them, with the increasing education of the consumer, the computerization of knowledge, and diminishing trust in professionals. Haug (1988) embellishes her assertions by highlighting the role of the mass media in popularizing medical knowledge. Similarly, Toren (1975) points to the potentially destabilizing influence on medicine and other professions of the growing standardization and routinization of knowledge. The more active engagement of the public in health issues in the United States than in Britain in terms of self-help, lobbying and litigation adds to the belief that the American medical profession may be in the process of decline. This belief is reinforced by the development, in new forms of managed care, of stronger consumer representation and complaint and grievance procedures, which provide greater opportunities for lay control (Weiss 1997). However, although such public involvement has had a negative impact on the professional powers of medicine, the consumer movement appears to have had less influence over the past two decades than the rising political leverage of business (Rodwin 1996). This is epitomized by the way in which advocacy groups themselves have often reinforced corporate interests in medical technology (Moran 1999).

In sum, then, for all the methodological difficulties involved, the medical profession seems to have been rather more affected by trends towards deprofessionalization in the United States than in Britain. Despite anti-trust action, deprofessionalization has not taken full effect because medicine has retained its collective monopolistic position and associated benefits, underwritten by state licensing laws (Freidson 1986). Doctors have also largely retained their prominent position in the labour force (Freidson 2001). This is highlighted by the considerable authority they still have over other health professions, as well as more immediate work tasks (Krause 1996), particularly as they have sought to make the system function in their interests (Light 1993). However, since the 1980s orthodox medicine seems to have lost some control of its work, not least through increasing supervision linked to the development of capitalism and the state. Whether this shift has engendered a growing sense of alienation is a moot point, but doctors have increasingly tended to form unions (McKinlay and Stoekle 1988). It is no longer possible, therefore, to argue that the medical profession is as dominant and autonomous as it ever was, especially in comparison with the pre-1970s era, when the fee-for-service system and doctor-controlled hospitals were the norm (Krause 1996). It is fascinating, though, that the deprofessionalization of medicine should now be being discussed in the Anglo-American context at the same time as the professionalization of previously marginalized alternative practitioners is gathering pace. It is to this trend that this chapter finally turns.

THE TREND TOWARDS THE PROFESSIONALIZATION OF ALTERNATIVE MEDICINE

Although not all alternative therapists are seeking to professionalize (see, for instance, Cant and Sharma 1995), the desirability of professionalization has grown for such practitioners in recent years. The reasons are varied. In Britain professionalization has been seen as providing protection against the increasing threat of harmonization within the European Union. This could result in more restrictive legislation governing the operation of alternative practitioners, abrogating their current common law rights in line with what happens in most other countries in Europe, where only orthodox health professionals are usually allowed to practise specific therapies (Huggon and Trench 1992). It has also carried the promise of enabling unorthodox therapists to cast off the stigmatizing labels of the past. Such promise has been most dramatically highlighted by the case of chiropractic in the United States, where its practitioners were officially able to shed the categorization of being 'unscientific' in the late 1980s – following a history of attacks on their legitimacy by the American Medical Association (Wardwell 1992). Professionalization based on exclusionary closure also has positive attractions from an interest viewpoint in terms of its more general potential to enhance income, status and power, as orthodox medicine has illustrated. This is over and above any satisfaction gained in ensuring that the therapies in question are well regulated in terms of benefiting the consumer in Britain and the United States (Saks 2000b).

THE PROFESSIONALIZATION OF ALTERNATIVE MEDICINE IN BRITAIN

Practitioners of alternative medicine have been described as being part of a 'holistic health movement' (Alster 1989). This concept, though, implies a cohesiveness that is belied by the considerable diversity that exists within unorthodox medicine – not least in the level of professionalization sought by different alternative therapies. Such diversity in Britain in fact thwarted the attempts of some groups of alternative practitioners to professionalize in the 1980s because the Conservative government of the day wished for a blanket approach that applied to all therapies (Sharma 1995). To be sure, a number of umbrella bodies existed, such as the Institute for Complementary Medicine, the Council for Complementary and Alternative Medicine and the British Complementary Medical Association. However, they were not able success-fully to bridge the divisions both within and between alternative therapies, including over the nature and scale of their professional aspirations (Fulder 1996). It was therefore with some relief to those alternative medical groups wishing to professionalize that the government abandoned its search for a unified approach in the early 1990s – leaving each therapy free to find its own place in terms of recognition (Sharma 1995).

The very broad spectrum of positions in relation to professionalization among unorthodox therapies in Britain is underlined by practices such as crystal therapy, which at present are strongly centred on self-help and have a less extensive knowledge base. Aromatherapy and reflexology are further along the path to professionalization, but are characterized by a wide range of occupational associations that have not yet fully come together – despite recent signs of progress (Mills and Budd 2000). Such fragmentation, together with the many training schools in existence, makes it very difficult to develop common standards for practitioners. The initial training involved, moreover, also tends to last for weeks and months, rather than years (Cant and Sharma 1995), and is therefore not the most powerful educational platform from which to launch claims for creating professional monopolies in the sense achieved by orthodox medicine. The acupuncturists and the homoeopaths, though, have moved their fields forward to a greater degree – albeit so far by establishing overarching mechanisms for voluntary self-regulation, as opposed to statutory regulation.

More specifically, non-medical acupuncturists have voluntarily put in place a unified code of discipline, education and ethics, to which most practitioners subscribe. This was achieved in 1980 after the founding of the Council for Acupuncture. It overcame the previous rifts between the British Acupuncture Association and Register, the Chung San Acupuncture Society, the Interna-tional Register of Oriental Medicine, the Register of Traditional Chinese Medicine and the Traditional Acupuncture Society. Self-regulatory arrange-ments were further developed with the formation of the British Acupuncture Accreditation Board, which established minimum educational standards, and the British Acupuncture Council, which acts as the registering body (Saks

1995a). In the case of homoeopathy, the Society of Homoeopaths has acted as the primary focus for the professionalization of the medically unqualified. Following its formation in 1981, the Society similarly established a voluntary register and laid down a code of ethics. Homoeopathy is not yet as unified as acupuncture; nonetheless, many homoeopathic colleges have now been officially accredited by the Society. In consequence, a recognized, systematic body of expertise has developed centred on a three-year full-time (or equivalent) education that provides a basis for further professional development (Cant and Sharma 1996).

However, after many years of campaigning, osteopathy and chiropractic have progressed their fields to a more advanced phase of professionalization – for which they have now obtained state support, through legislation passed in the first half of the 1990s. The internal splits within osteopathy were sufficiently reconciled for the 1993 Osteopathy Act to enter the statute book. This established the General Osteopathic Council, the main role of which is to oversee a register that has been formed to uphold ethical and educational standards and give statutory protection of title (Standen 1993). The parallel 1994 Chiropractic Act that followed this legislation is based on the standards of education and practice of the British Chiropractic Association, which most chiropractors felt able to accept. It too provides for state registration, pivoted in this case on the founding of the General Chiropractic Council (Cant and Sharma 1995). But while the two pieces of legislation represent a major watershed for alternative medicine in terms of professionalization based on exclusionary closure in Britain, there are limits to the legal monopolies gained. Most notably, they do not provide privileged access to practice in the National Health Service, as state underwriting has done for more orthodox health professions. Despite mainstream acceptance, therefore, there are still real restrictions on the funding on which the new professions can draw.

THE PROFESSIONALIZATION OF ALTERNATIVE MEDICINE IN THE UNITED STATES

It should be reiterated at this point that the process of professionalization of alternative medicine has moved at an even greater pace in the United States. The degree of professionalization is accentuated by the example of osteopathy discussed in Chapter 4, which – as in Britain – was originally heavily attacked by the medical profession. It was noted there that osteopaths were gradually incorporated into medicine itself in a long process going back several decades (Gevitz 1988a). This culminated in their licensing as professional equals across a range of American states by the 1960s and 1970s, which in practice made them eligible for medical residencies, certification as medical specialists and appointments to the staff of medical hospitals (Wardwell 1994a). Before the Osteopathy Act was passed in Britain, Baer (1987: 64) commented on the comparative position of American osteopaths as follows: 'Whereas osteopathy has become osteopathic medicine and osteopaths have become osteopathic physicians in the United States, in many ways osteopathy in Britain resembles what it looked like in the United States perhaps sixty or seventy years ago.' The position has clearly changed with the passage of the 1993 Act, but this quotation clearly highlights that whereas American osteopaths are now consolidating and extending their professional standing, those in Britain have only just won their professional spurs.

The case of chiropractic illustrates that the professionalization of alternative medicine has also been accelerated in other fields over the past two or three decades in the United States. As previously documented, chiropractors have now gained widespread state licensure, as well as the right to reimbursement under Medicare and Medicaid. Admittedly, there are variations between states in the breadth and focus of the statutory parameters within which chiropractors work – including whether they are permitted to sign death certificates, to carry out school examinations, and to practise in such areas as obstetrics and naturopathy (Wardwell 1994b). However, they do now formally have professional standing. As we have seen, a court ruling in the late 1980s that required the American Medical Association to end its boycott of chiropractic reinforced this position. The practical effect of the ruling was to give chiropractors, among other things, professional consultation rights with doctors and access to diagnostic facilities in medical hospitals (Wardwell 1994a). The outcome reflected the tactics of the chiropractors in their long-running attempts to professionalize, in which they had proclaimed their 'scientific' expertise, established lengthy education programmes and increased the research underpinning of their practice (Martin 1994).

Just as in Britain, though, not all alternative therapies have moved in the direction of professionalization. The largest use of such therapies in the United States – following the case of Britain – continues to be based on self-help, as opposed to practitioner-centred delivery (Eisenberg et al. 1998). It may therefore not be appropriate for professionalization to be contemplated in every field of unorthodox therapy in terms of the knowledge and skills involved. As in Britain too, there are a myriad of occupational associations representing each therapy. In acupuncture, for example, these bodies range from the American Association of Acupuncture and Bio-energetic Medicine to the American Association of Acupuncture and Oriental Medicine (Bruce and McIlwain 1998). Licensing in such fields is typically based on graduation from accredited schools in the therapy concerned. In acupuncture, bodies such as the National Council of Acupuncture Schools and Colleges and the National Commission for the Certification of Acupuncturists underwrite the authenticity of the qualifications obtained. Such arrangements are paralleled in other areas. Thus in naturopathy, for instance, the Council on Naturopathic Medical Education is pivotal (Cohen 1998).

In contrast to Britain, however, the form of the licensing of naturopathy, acupuncture and other alternative therapies varies from state to state in the more decentralized political system of the United States, and therefore depends on local judgements (Bruce and McIlwain 1998). Even the existence of licensing for particular therapies – which usually brings with it exclusivity of practice and self-regulatory obligations – is not universal. Whereas acupuncture is licensed in the majority of states, for example, naturopathy is similarly underwritten only in just over a dozen. This variation is also highlighted by the case of massage therapy. While this is licensed in about half of the states, the examination of the National Certification Board for Therapeutic Massage and Bodywork is adopted by only half of these again. Intriguingly, too, the scope of practice and even the basic legislative definition of apparently the same therapy can fluctuate between states (Cohen 1998). This all adds up to a disjointed patchwork of professionalization of specific alternative therapies in the United States, which extends to some states, but not all. Importantly, in many cases the medical profession remains in control. This is illustrated by the case of acupuncture, which, as previously noted, is defined in most states as a medical modality suitable for practice only under the authority of a physician (Saks 1995b).

Mention of orthodox biomedicine raises the question of whether the professionalization of alternative medicine is necessarily desirable from the viewpoint of state health policy in Britain and the United States. One issue – which may explain why some alternative practitioners do not find professionalization an attractive concept – is whether it creates barriers that conflict with the holistic, egalitarian philosophies of some forms of unorthodox medicine. The more alternative therapists are drawn into an institutional role in surveillance and control through state and/or private corporate sponsorship (Saks 2000b), the more such barriers are likely to form. As we have seen, there are also other downsides to professionalization, as the case of medicine underlines – not least being the way in which such enclaves of exclusionary social closure can become pockets of self-interested protectionism that retard progress, despite the positive ideologies of professional bodies. Indeed, it is the public backlash against such protectionism that has partly threatened the deprofessionalization of medicine in the wake of the rise of a strong counter-culture, as discussed in Chapter 4. In this regard, from an interest perspective, the growing professionalization of alternative medicine has accentuated the challenge to mainstream medicine by legitimating potential competitors both to the increasing number of orthodox exponents of such therapies and to those exclusively practising biomedicine.

On the other hand, the professionalization of alternative therapies may serve to increase collaboration between orthodox and alternative practitioners by reducing uncertainty about the quality of the service provided and standardizing what can be expected from alternative therapists. This reduction of uncertainty can be very important in facilitating cooperation, especially given the dangers of litigation consequent on referral and delegation, where the doctor remains accountable for the care of the patient (Stone and Mathews 1996). The mutual benefits are also well illustrated by the relief that alternative therapists can provide from repeat visits to general practitioners by chronically ill patients for whom they can do little in the British context (Peters 1994). They are highlighted too by the professional incorporation of osteopaths in the United States, which helped the medical profession to fill its many intern vacancies. This was facilitated by a trade-off between the professional recognition of the osteopaths for control over their supply and the creation of a biomedical knowledge base (Blackstone 1977). The advantages to the consumer of professionalization lie primarily in the educational, ethical and research framework that has typically been developed by specific alternative therapies as part of the process of becoming a profession. This framework can provide greater protection to clients of unorthodox practitioners, particularly when safety, efficacy and cost are key issues (Saks 2000b). This discussion leads neatly on to the likely relationship of orthodox and alternative medicine in the Anglo-American context in the future, which is considered in the Conclusion.

Conclusion

The development of orthodox and alternative medicine, and the links between them, has now been examined over several centuries in Britain and the United States. The book has therefore run most of its compelling course. It has moved from studying the period when the distinction between these two spheres did not yet exist, to considering the time when they became very starkly polarized. It has also explored the most recent signs of some kind of *rapprochement* between orthodox and alternative medicine, following the emergence of a strong counter-culture. This volume has sought to highlight the political dimensions of this process, especially those related to self-interests – defined in this context in terms of advancing the income, status and power of the groups involved. The notion of professionalization based on exclusionary closure has been central to the analysis, given its key role in the marginalization of alternative medicine by medical orthodoxy and paradoxically now in the resurgence of unorthodox therapies. A number of associated issues have also been discussed. These include why orthodox medicine was initially able to professionalize, the reasons for the subsequent marginalization of unorthodox therapies, how far the deprofessionalization of conventional medicine is currently in train and the extent to which the professionalization of alternative medicine has occurred in the Anglo-American context.

The analysis suggests that the further integration of orthodox and alternative medicine could bring great benefit to the consumer. In looking to the future, therefore, the Conclusion focuses on how this may be achieved. Such benefit is most likely to result if the best of the current range of orthodox medical practices are employed, along with the complementary strengths of the increasingly popular and even more diverse span of alternative therapies. As we have seen, the latter may be most helpful in dealing with areas such as chronic illness, in which orthodox biomedicine has less to offer, for all its other achievements. Moreover, although alternative therapies are often more labour-intensive – with consultations usually lasting considerably longer than those with primary care physicians – the costs of the remedies and technologies involved are typically much lower (Saks 1994). This lower cost represents an added advantage over orthodox medicine at a time when cost containment is a key issue. It was also noted earlier that some types of alternative therapies are attractive because of their comparative safety, reflecting their characteristic emphasis on the promotion of health rather than simply the treatment of illness (Fulder 1996). In all these respects, it is important that the forms of orthodox and alternative medicine for which there is substantial contrary evidence are discarded – and that the therapies for which there is the most significant positive support are embraced.

Thus there is a need for decisions about 'best practice' to be underpinned by research. The concept of 'evidence-based' practice brings to the fore the question of what is to count as the 'best' of both worlds, especially given the methodological disputes that have long raged about the most appropriate means of evaluating alternative, as opposed to orthodox, medicine in Britain and the United States. These throw into focus the issue of how central the randomized controlled trial should be in assessing such therapies. This may not be easy to resolve, as they are often rooted in methodological assumptions incommensurable with biomedicine, based on the individual nature of the treatments given and with a greater emphasis placed on qualitative outcomes (Saks 1998a). As noted in the Introduction, it may therefore be necessary to go beyond rigid claims about the 'objective' scientific status of orthodox medicine and acknowledge that the rules of the methodological game are far from universal. Orthodox and alternative medicine could then be brought together in the most productive manner – taking into account not only the relative strengths and weaknesses of particular therapies, but also how they may be best delivered in practice.

From the viewpoint of the delivery of such therapies in the Anglo-American context, there are many possible organizational frameworks. Leaving aside the employment of orthodox and unorthodox medicine on a self-help basis, these raise a number of important questions. Should specific alternative therapies be applied in mainstream health contexts, in completely separate settings, or as part of a new integrated service based on holistic health centres? Should physicians be the gatekeepers for alternative therapies or should orthodox and alternative practitioners operate as co-equals, working alongside each other? Should alternative practitioners generally seek the legally enshrined professional regulatory frameworks possessed by orthodox health professionals? Should all fields of unorthodox practice be at least minimally based on the establishment of codes of ethics and lengthy education programmes, even if they do not gain formal exclusionary closure? Should shared learning with conventional practitioners be encouraged, in order to enhance future collaboration, and if so at what level? How, moreover, should the development of an evidence base be supported for alternative therapies – by the private sector, the state, or both, as in the case of orthodox medicine? And who should pay for the therapies concerned – the consumer at the point of access, the insurance plans, or the state? While the resolution of such issues is in part value based, it must again be informed by research (Best and Glik 2000).

Some of these issues were discussed at a specially convened conference held in 2001 entitled 'Can Alternative Medicine Be Integrated into Mainstream Care?', jointly organized by the Royal College of Physicians in Britain and the National Center for Complementary and Alternative Medicine in the United States. The very title of the conference suggests that one of the key difficulties in enhancing integration may be the interest of orthodox medicine in controlling alternative therapies. It has been emphasized in this book that it should not necessarily be assumed that professional groups serve the public interest, as opposed to their own self-interests, despite the prevailing ideologies of professions. While moves to incorporate alternative therapies into conventional medicine are now under way in both Britain and the United States, some contributors fear that these may result in a form of integration excessively skewed towards biomedicine. In this regard, Cant and Sharma (1999) note that 'integration' may become synonymous with the medical 'appropriation' of alternative therapies at the expense of the public. This threat is linked to the continuing dominance of medical interests in health care. Although this may have declined in recent years – albeit rather more in the United States than in Britain – it remains a significant issue for the future.

In terms of balance, it is also important to note the potential detrimental impact of the competing interests of groups of alternative practitioners, who may themselves be seeking parochially to ensure their own ascendancy, in the face of the long-term dominance of medicine (Saks 2001). In this respect, it could be argued that a cautious approach to integration, placing it under the wing of orthodox medicine, is advisable to protect the public from undue risk. Such an approach may be justified if substantial harm is likely to be caused by alternative practitioners, particularly where they have little or no knowledge of biomedicine and/or the therapies that they are purveying. This danger is receding, though, with the growing professionalization of alternative medicine (Saks 2000b). On the other hand, the many orthodox health professionals whose patients do not feel sufficiently confident to tell them when they are using unorthodox therapies pose a threat to the public (Cohen 1998). So may orthodox health professionals practising alternative medicine who are trained to a lower standard than non-medically qualified therapists. There are also risks when such personnel lack the knowledge to make sensible referrals to alternative therapists (Cant and Sharma 1999). The extent to which doctors and allied health professionals can operate without sanction in the current manner may itself reflect ongoing medical hegemony.

If entrenched professional interests primarily sustain the current position, major catalysts for change may be necessary for integration in health care to be enhanced in the Anglo-American context. One such catalyst in Britain has been the high-profile report on *Integrated Healthcare*, produced by the Foundation for Integrated Medicine (1997), under the sponsorship of the Prince of Wales. This was designed to prompt consideration of the way forward for the next five years as a spur to government action. It was based on the reports of four working groups that made sensitive and inclusive proposals for advancing the agenda in relation to research and development, education and training, regulation, and delivery mechanisms. In the United States, the direction of work on alternative medicine has also been positively affected by publications such as *Manifesto for a New Medicine*, produced by the first chair of the Advisory Council of the Office of Alternative Medicine (Gordon 1996). In the more devolved American political system, this book focuses on small-scale case studies that show how orthodox medicine can be synthesized with alternative therapies at grassroots level. Its aim is to provide a guide to healing partnerships and the wise use of alternative medicine, to facilitate more effective integration with biomedicine through the consumer.

The intervention of the federal state, however, is now likely to have the most critical influence on this field. In this respect, two recent national initiatives in the Anglo-American context hold much promise in developing further the *rapprochement* between orthodox and alternative medicine. In Britain the driving force has been the report by the House of Lords Select Committee on Science and Technology (2000) on complementary and alternative medicine. Drawing on evidence submitted from many interested parties, this report makes a threefold distinction between complementary and alternative therapies. The first group delineated by the Committee is composed of acupuncture, chiropractic, herbal medicine, homoeopathy and osteopathy. These therapies are centred on individual diagnosis and treatment, and are seen to possess the most credible evidence base and the most organized groups of practitioners. The second group of therapies, exemplified by aromatherapy, counselling, hypnotherapy, massage and reflexology, are held to complement conventional medicine. The defining feature of the third group is felt to be that the therapies concerned have philosophical principles counterposed to those of mainstream medicine, as well as the weakest research base. This group encompasses such long-established health systems as Ayurvedic Medicine and Traditional Chinese Medicine, together with crystal therapy, iridology and radionics.

On the basis of these distinctions, the report makes a number of recommendations to government, most of which have been well received (Department of Health 2001b). Among these are the following:

- The National Health Service should ensure access to complementary and alternative therapies through medical referral where there is evidence of efficacy and/or robust regulatory mechanisms.
- Single professional regulatory structures should be developed for such therapies, on a statutory or voluntary basis as appropriate.
- Training in their practice should be linked to higher education, encompassing where relevant an understanding of research methods as well as biomedical knowledge.
- Orthodox health professions should be more systematically familiarized with complementary and alternative medicine and draw up guidelines on standards for their members.
- Research into complementary and alternative medicine should be extended, with pump-priming monies from government.
- More information about such therapies should be made available to the public, not least through the National Health Service helpline NHS Direct.

The document echoes some of the recommendations of earlier reports, including that of the British Medical Association (1993), while providing its own distinctive gloss. One key difference from the latter report is that it adopts a more eclectic view of research methods and argues for ring-fenced research funding for non-conventional medicine.

Although the House of Lords Select Committee report has been criticized – not least for the apparent inconsistency of placing acupuncture in group 1 of its categorization, while locating Traditional Chinese Medicine in group 3 – it has undoubtedly moved the field forward in Britain. In America, its work has been paralleled by that of the White House Commission, which was established in 2000 by President Clinton to report on complementary and alternative medicine because of the high level of public interest in, and use of, unorthodox medicine (National Center for Complementary and Alternative Medicine 2001b). The Commission was tasked with making recommendations to the President of the United States to ensure that public policy maximizes the benefits of such therapies. The final report of the *White House Commission on Complementary and Alternative Medicine Policy* (2002) has now been published, following extensive consultation with many stakeholders. It includes such proposals as:

- The Department of Health and Human Services should develop strategies for increasing consumer access to safe and effective forms of complementary and alternative medicine.
- An office should be created to coordinate federal complementary and

alternative medicine activities and facilitate their integration into the national health care system.

- Insurers and managed care organizations should offer purchasers the option of health benefit plans incorporating appropriate complementary and alternative medicine interventions.
- The education and training of both complementary and alternative medicine and orthodox medical practitioners should be designed to ensure public safety and improve health.
- The dialogue between complementary and alternative medicine practitioners and conventional medical professionals should be strengthened.
- The federal, private and non-profit sectors should support more research into complementary and alternative medicine, which needs a stronger research infrastructure.
- The federal government and the states should ensure that accurate, useful and easily accessible information is available on complementary and alternative medicine.

Leaving aside the references to the distinctive American political context, there are clearly many resonances with the recommendations of the report of the House of Lords Select Committee on Science and Technology (2000), on which the Commission explicitly draws.

The importance of federal involvement in the development of alternative medicine in the United States, in addition to the efforts made to integrate it with orthodox medicine in individual states (Cohen 1998), is also highlighted by the progress that has been made through the National Center for Complementary and Alternative Medicine. This body, which is part of the National Institutes of Health, is anticipating further budget increases under the Bush administration from the $89 million it received in fiscal year 2001, following low-level beginnings in its previous form as the Office of Alternative Medicine in the early 1990s. Its high-priority areas of research range from investigating the mechanisms of complementary and alternative medicine to facilitating the successful integration of safe and effective non-conventional therapies into mainstream medicine (National Center for Complementary and Alternative Medicine 2001a). The Center also throws up a dilemma related to enhanced government involvement in complementary and alternative medicine – namely, that, as the level of investment rises, the field may be subject to ever-greater biomedical capture. This is in part because escalating federal funding provides interest-based incentives for orthodox doctors and medical researchers to enter this area, which may work to the prejudice of a balanced pattern of integration in health care.

The experience of other Western countries also points the way to a more integrated future in health care. In continental Europe the contemporary growth in popularity of alternative medicine has broadly mirrored that in Britain. This has led to its expanding use by health professionals, as well as increasing support from the state (Fisher and Ward 1994). Unlike in Britain, governments in many other European countries adhere to traditional legal codes that restrict the practice of alternative medicine to registered medical professionals. However, in the light of increasing public interest in such therapies, a number of governments have allowed the expansion of practice beyond existing medical bounds. As early as 1970 in the Netherlands, for example, the State Commission on Medical Practice recommended that the medically unqualified should be prevented from practising alternative medicine only where public health was at risk (Fulder 1996). The extent of state interest in alternative therapies in Europe more generally is highlighted by the recent 5-year Cooperation in Science and Technology project on unconventional medicine, sponsored by the European Commission. This project involved researchers from Belgium, Croatia, Denmark, Finland, Germany, Hungary, Italy, the Netherlands, Norway, Slovenia, Spain, Sweden and Switzerland, as well as Britain. Its aim was 'to foster international collaboration in research into the therapeutic significance of unconventional medicine, its cost–benefit ratio and its socio-cultural importance as a basis for evaluation of its possible usefulness or risks in public health' (Monckton *et al.* 1998: 8).

From a North American perspective, there has been progress towards integrated health care in Canada too. Kelner and Wellman (1997b) document how alternative medicine is flourishing alongside orthodox biomedicine – in a system where patients choose the type of practitioner that they believe will best help their specific problem. While there is variation between the provinces/territories in the official provision made for alternative therapies (Clarke 1990), at a national level increasing priority is being placed on people-focused services. The same priority is evident in the more consumer-oriented systems of managed care in Canada. As in the United States, therefore, growing attention has been given to integrating orthodox and alternative medicine for the benefit of the consumer – including by enhancing health information services, improving funding for health research, and supporting self-care and prevention across these fields (Best and Glik 2000). In this spirit, Health Canada established an Advisory Group on Complementary and Alternative Health Care in 1999 to identify crucial health system issues and propose a future strategy (Shearer and Simpson 2001). It also set up an Office of Natural Health Products to help ensure that alternative medicine is effective, safe and of high quality, while respecting the individual rights and diversity of Canada's population (De Bruyn 2001). However, as in Europe and the United States, such an approach will not bring about positive changes in the extent of integrated health care without multi-sectoral collaboration and bottom-up thinking (Best and Glik 2000).

This point is underlined in countries in the East such as China and India, where therapies that are regarded as alternative medicine today in Britain and the United States are more strongly embedded as part of orthodox medicine, alongside biomedicine which has spread from the West (Saks 1997b). In China, for example, there are many hundreds of thousands of practitioners of the long-standing system of Traditional Chinese Medicine, and all hospitals have an outpatient clinic for traditional medicine (Fulder 1996). This contrasts with its relative marginality in the Anglo-American context. That said, even in China exponents of Traditional Chinese Medicine do not necessarily operate on a level playing field with their orthodox counterparts, given the current popularity of Western biomedicine. Indeed, they were formally banned in the past – as when Traditional Chinese Medicine, with its characteristic *yin–yang* philosophy, was suppressed in the 1920s by the Kuomintang, because it was seen as running counter to the modernization of China (Saks 1995b). Acupuncture, herbal remedies and other aspects of this form of health care, however, were revived following the Communist Revolution in 1949, and now both Traditional Chinese Medicine and biomedicine receive strong state support (Bray 2000). Thus the alternatives of today can become the orthodoxy of tomorrow – thereby underscoring the fluidity of the boundary between orthodox and alternative medicine.

Given the impact of philosophies from the East on the development of the contemporary counter-culture in the West in the 1960s and 1970s, it is tempting to see the integration that is presently emerging primarily as a fusion of Eastern alternatives and Western biomedicine. In practice, though, the situation is much more complex. To be sure, Eastern philosophies have greatly influenced both Britain and the United States. Such influence is well exemplified by the books of Deepak Chopra, which have sold many millions of copies and aim to help readers to increase their energy levels using Ayurvedic principles (see, for instance, Chopra 1995). These principles underpin much of the traditional health care in the Indian subcontinent (Cant and Sharma 1999). They hold that individuals have varying body types with differing amounts of *vata*, *pitta* and *kapha* that influence, among other things, movement, digestion and the balance of bodily fluids. As we have seen, however, there are also many indigenous influences on alternative medicine in the Anglo-American context. These are illustrated by chiropractic and osteopathy, which were founded in the United States, and the distinctly British herbal heritage that runs alongside that of China and India (Fulder 1996). In addition, it should again be stressed that when therapies such as acupuncture have been adopted in the West, they have frequently been transformed into biomedical modalities that bear little resemblance to their ancient practice in the East (Saks 1995b).

These international examples indicate that the future pattern of integration of orthodox and alternative medicine in Britain and the United States is likely largely to reflect the particular history and socio-political context of each of these societies (Saks 1997b). In Europe and North America the popularity of specific alternative therapies varies from country to country, partly related to cultural preferences. In France, for instance, the most widely used therapy is homoeopathy, whereas in the Netherlands it is spiritual healing and in Denmark reflexology (Fisher and Ward 1994). Interestingly, the latter two therapies do not figure as strongly in Britain as practices such as acupuncture and herbal medicine. In Canada, meanwhile, chiropractic is the most popular type of alternative medicine – with chiropractors now constituting the third biggest group of primary care practitioners after doctors and dentists. While there is a similar pattern in the United States, Canada is distinguished by the greater degree of prominence given to naturopathy (Clarke 1990). It should be noted that professional interests have also been important influences in shaping the terrain. In France, for instance, homoeopathy has flourished largely because by law its use is exclusively restricted to physicians (Fulder 1996), which has effectively eliminated competition and opened up the field for colonization by medical orthodoxy.

This is a reminder that the nature and form of integration of orthodox and alternative medicine vary across nations – and that it is not always the non-medically qualified who are the standard-bearers for alternative therapies. It underlines too that the extent to which integration occurs is affected by a wide range of factors. These range from the degree of compatibility of the philosophies underlying particular orthodox and alternative therapies to 'belief barriers' in orthodox medicine about the acceptance of non-conventional health care (Cohen 1998). As has been indicated, the specific conjunction of occupational self-interests in the health field may well be one of the most significant ingredients in this equation. This has been a central theme of this volume, as part of the neo-Weberian analysis of the politics of professionalization in Britain and the United States. The author hopes that this analysis will enable the main field-breaking aim of this book to be realized – that is, to provide a rounded social scientific account of the historical, contemporary and possible future development of health care in the Anglo-American context, which recognizes that orthodox and alternative medicine are two seamlessly interrelated sides of the same coin.

References

Abel-Smith, B. (1960) *A History of the Nursing Profession*, London: Heinemann.

Abel-Smith, B. (1976) *Value for Money in Health Services*, London: Heinemann.

Acheson, D. (1998) *Independent Inquiry into Inequalities in Health*, London: HMSO.

Aday, L., Andersen, R. and Fleming, G. (1980) *Health Care in the United States: Equitable for Whom?*, Beverly Hills, CA: Sage.

Alaszewski, A. (1995) 'Restructuring health and welfare professions in the United Kingdom: the impact of internal markets on the medical, nursing and social work professions', in Johnson, T., Larkin, G. and Saks, M. (eds) *Health Professions and the State in Europe*, London: Routledge.

Allsop, J. (1995a) *Health Policy and the NHS*, 2nd edition, London: Longman.

Allsop, J. (1995b) 'Shifting spheres of opportunity: the professional powers of general practitioners within the British National Health Service', in Johnson, T., Larkin, G. and Saks, M. (eds) *Health Professions and the State in Europe*, London: Routledge.

Allsop, J. (1999) 'Identity maintenance under conditions of change: the medical profession in the late twentieth century', in Hellberg, I., Saks, M. and Benoit, C. (eds) *Professional Identities in Transition: Cross-cultural Dimensions*, Södertälje, Sweden: Almqvist & Wiksell International.

Allsop, J. and Mulcahy, L. (1996) *Regulating Medical Work: Formal and Informal Controls*, Buckingham: Open University Press.

Allsop, J. and Mulcahy, L. (1999) 'Doctors' responses to patient complaints', in Rosenthal, M., Mulcahy, L. and Lloyd-Bostock, S. (eds) *Medical Mishaps: Pieces of the Puzzle*, Buckingham: Open University Press.

Alster, K. (1989) *The Holistic Health Movement*, Tuscaloosa: University of Alabama Press.

Alternative Medicine: Expanding Medical Horizons (1994) Report to the National Institutes of Health on Alternative Medical Systems and Practices in the United States, Washington, DC: US Government Printing Office.

American Medical Association (1912) *Nostrums and Quackery*, vol. 1, Chicago: AMA.

American Medical Association (1921) *Nostrums and Quackery*, vol. 2, Chicago: AMA.

Anderson, O. (1989) 'Issues in the health services of the United States', in Field, M. G. (ed.) *Success and Crisis in National Health Systems*, London: Routledge.

Annandale, E. (1998) *The Sociology of Health and Medicine: A Critical Introduction*, Cambridge: Polity Press.

Ashton, J. and Seymour, H. (1990) *The New Public Health*, Buckingham: Open University Press.

Astin, J. (2000) 'The characteristics of CAM users: a complex picture', in Kelner, M., Wellman, B., Pescosolido, B. and Saks, M. (eds) *Complementary and Alternative Medicine: Challenge and Change*, Amsterdam: Harwood Academic Publishers.

Baer, H. (1987) 'The divergent evolution of osteopathy in America and Britain', in Roth, J. (ed.) *Research in the Sociology of Health Care*, vol. 5, Greenwich, CT: JAI Press.

Baggott, R. (2000) *Public Health: Policy and Politics*, Basingstoke: Macmillan.

Bakx, K. (1991) 'The "eclipse" of folk medicine in Western society', *Sociology of Health and Illness*, 13: 20–38.

Barber, B. (1963) 'Some problems in the sociology of professions', *Daedalus*, 92: 669–88.

Barry, J. (1987) 'Publicity and the public good: presenting medicine in eighteenth century Bristol', in Bynum, W. F. and Porter, R. (eds) *Medical Fringe and Medical Orthodoxy 1750–1850*, London: Croom Helm.

Bartrip, P. (1990) *Mirror of Medicine: A History of the BMJ*, Oxford: Clarendon Press.

Baucher, H. (2001) 'What's up (or down and out) in US healthcare', *Archives of Disease in Childhood*, 85: 11.

Berlant, J. L. (1975) *Profession and Monopoly: A Study of Medicine in the United States and Great Britain*, Berkeley: University of California Press.

Berliner, H. S. (1985a) *A System of Scientific Medicine: Philanthropic Foundations in the Flexner Era*, London: Tavistock.

Berliner, H. S. (1985b) 'Scientific medicine since Flexner', in Salmon, J. W. (ed.) *Alternative Medicines: Popular and Policy Perspectives*, London: Tavistock.

Bertens, H. (1995) *The Idea of the Postmodern: A History*, London: Routledge.

Best, A. and Glik, D. (2000) 'Research as a tool for integrative health services reform', in Kelner, M., Wellman, B., Pescosolido, B. and Saks, M. (eds)

Complementary and Alternative Medicine: Challenge and Change, Amsterdam: Harwood Academic Publishers.

Blackstone, E. (1977) 'The AMA and the osteopaths: a study of the power of organized medicine', *Antitrust Bulletin,* 22: 405–40.

Blondel, J. (1995) *Comparative Government: An Introduction,* Hemel Hempstead: Prentice Hall/Harvester Wheatsheaf.

Blume, S. (2000) 'Medicine, technology and industry', in Cooter, R. and Pickstone, J. (eds) *Medicine in the Twentieth Century,* Amsterdam: Harwood Academic Publishers.

Bodenheimer, T. (1985) 'The transnational pharmaceutical industry and the health of the world's people', in McKinlay, J. (ed.) *Issues in the Political Economy of Health Care,* London: Tavistock.

Botelho, R. (2000) 'The UK healthcare renaissance: a transatlantic perspective', *Journal of Interprofessional Care,* 14: 87–93.

Brandt, A. and Gardner, M. (2000) 'The golden age of medicine?', in Cooter, R. and Pickstone, J. (eds) *Medicine in the Twentieth Century,* Amsterdam: Harwood Academic Publishers.

Brannon, R. L. (1996) 'Restructuring hospital nursing: reversing the trend toward a professional work force', *International Journal of Health Services,* 26: 643–54.

Bray, F. (2000) 'The Chinese experience', in Cooter, R. and Pickstone, J. (eds) *Medicine in the Twentieth Century,* Amsterdam: Harwood Academic Publishers.

Brazier, M., Lovecy, J., Moran, M. and Potton, M. (1993) 'Falling from a tightrope: doctors and lawyers between the market and the state', *Political Studies,* 61: 197–213.

British Medical Association (1909) *Secret Remedies: What They Cost and What They Contain,* London: BMA.

British Medical Association (1912) *More Secret Remedies,* London: BMA.

British Medical Association (1986) *Report of the Board of Science and Education on Alternative Therapy,* London: BMA.

British Medical Association (1993) *Complementary Medicine: New Approaches to Good Practice,* London: BMA.

British Medical Association (2000) *Acupuncture: Efficacy, Safety and Practice,* Amsterdam: Harwood Academic Publishers.

Britten, N. (1996) 'Lay views of drugs and medicines: orthodox and unorthodox accounts', in Williams, S. and Calnan, M. (eds) *Modern Medicine: Lay Perspectives and Experiences,* London: UCL Press.

Brown, E. R. (1979) *Rockefeller Medicine Men: Capitalism and Medical Care in America,* Berkeley: University of California Medical Press.

Brown, P. S. (1985) 'The vicissitudes of herbalism in late nineteenth and early twentieth century Britain', *Medical History,* 29: 71–92.

Brown, P. S. (1987) 'Social context and medical theory in the demarcation of nineteenth-century boundaries', in Bynum, W. F. and Porter, R. (eds) *Medical Fringe and Medical Orthodoxy 1750–1850*, London: Croom Helm.

Bruce, D. F. and McIlwain, H. H. (1998) *The Unofficial Guide to Alternative Medicine*, New York: Macmillan.

Bunker, J. (1997) 'Ivan Illich and the pursuit of health', *Journal of Health Services Research and Policy*, 2: 56–9.

Burrow, J. G. (1963) *AMA: Voice of American Medicine*, Baltimore: Johns Hopkins Press.

Busfield, J. (2000) *Health and Health Care in Modern Britain*, Oxford: Oxford University Press.

Butler, J. and Vaile, M. (1984) *Health and Health Services: An Introduction to Health Care in Britain*, London: Routledge & Kegan Paul.

Bynum, W. F. (1987) 'Treating the wages of sin: venereal disease and specialism in eighteenth century England', in Bynum, W. F. and Porter, R. (eds) *Medical Fringe and Medical Orthodoxy 1750–1850*, London: Croom Helm.

Bynum, W. F. (1994) *Science and the Practice of Medicine in the Nineteenth Century*, Cambridge: Cambridge University Press.

Cant, S. and Sharma, U. (1995) *Professionalisation in Complementary Medicine*. Report on a research project funded by the Economic and Social Research Council.

Cant, S. and Sharma, U. (1996) 'Demarcation and transformation within homoeopathic knowledge: a strategy of professionalization', *Social Science and Medicine*, 42: 579–88.

Cant, S. and Sharma, U. (1999) *A New Medical Pluralism? Alternative Medicine, Doctors, Patients and the State*, London: UCL Press.

Chandler, J. (1996) 'The United States', in Wall, A. (ed.) *Health Care Systems in Liberal Democracies*, London: Routledge.

Chopra, D. (1995) *Boundless Energy*, London: Ryder.

Clarke, J. (1990) *Health, Illness and Medicine in Canada*, Toronto: McClelland & Stewart.

Coburn, D. (1999) 'Professions in transition: globalisation, neo-liberalism and the decline of medical power', in Hellberg, I., Saks, M. and Benoit, C. (eds) *Professional Identities in Transition: Cross-cultural Dimensions*, Södertälje: Almqvist & Wiksell International.

Coburn, D. and Biggs, L. (1986) 'Limits to medical dominance: the case of chiropractic', *Social Science and Medicine*, 22: 1035–46.

Cohen, M. (1998) *Complementary and Alternative Medicine: Legal Boundaries and Regulatory Perspectives*, Baltimore: Johns Hopkins University Press.

Collins, R. (1990) 'Market closure and the conflict theory of the professions', in Burrage, M. and Torstendahl, R. (eds) *Professions in Theory and History: Rethinking the Study of the Professions*, London: Sage.

Colombotos, J. (1969) ' Physicians and Medicare: a before–after study of the effect of legislation on attitudes', *American Sociological Review*, 34: 318–34.

Coward, R. (1989) *The Whole Truth: The Myth of Alternative Medicine*, London: Faber & Faber.

Cox, D. (1991) 'Health service management – a sociological view: Griffiths and the non-negotiated order of the hospital', in Gabe, J., Calnan, M. and Bury, M. (eds) *The Sociology of the Health Service*, London: Routledge.

Crompton, R. (1990) 'Professions in the current context', *Work, Employment and Society*, Special Issue: 147–66.

Cule, J. (1997) 'The history of medicine: from its ancient origins to the modern world', in Porter, R. (ed.) *Medicine: A History of Healing*, London: Ivy Press.

Dally, A. (1997) 'The development of Western medical science', in Porter, R. (ed.) *Medicine: A History of Healing*, London: Ivy Press.

Davies, C. (1999) 'Rethinking regulation in the health professions in the UK: institutions, ideals and identities', in Hellberg, I., Saks, M. and Benoit, C. (eds) *Professional Identities in Transition: Cross-cultural Dimensions*, Södertälje, Sweden: Almqvist & Wiksell International.

Davies, C. and Beach, A. (2000) *Interpreting Professional Self-Regulation: A History of the United Kingdom Central Council for Nursing, Midwifery and Health Visiting*, London: Routledge.

Davies, C., Finlay, L. and Bullman, A. (eds) (2000) *Changing Practice in Health and Social Care*, London: Sage.

De Bruyn, T. (2001) 'Taking stock: policy issues associated with complementary and alternative health care', in Shearer, R. and Simpson, J. (eds) *Perspectives on Complementary and Alternative Health Care*, Ottawa: Health Canada.

Department of Health (1989) *Working for Patients*, London: HMSO.

Department of Health (1991) *The Patient's Charter*, London: HMSO.

Department of Health (1992) *The Health of the Nation*, London: HMSO.

Department of Health (1997) *The New NHS: Modern, Dependable*, London: HMSO.

Department of Health (1998) *Our Healthier Nation: A Contract for Health*, London: HMSO.

Department of Health (1999) *Saving Lives: Our Healthier Nation*, London: HMSO.

Department of Health (2000a) *A Health Service of All the Talents: Developing the NHS Workforce*, London: Department of Health.

Department of Health (2000b) *Research and Development for a First Class Service*, London: Department of Health.

Department of Health (2000c) *The NHS Plan*, London: The Stationery Office.

Department of Health (2001a) *Establishing the New Nursing and Midwifery Council*, London: Department of Health.

Department of Health (2001b) *Government Response to the House of Lords Select Committee on Science and Technology's Report on Complementary and Alternative Medicine*, London: The Stationery Office.

Department of Health (2001c) *Modernising Regulation in the Health Professions*, London: Department of Health.

Department of Health (2001d) *Modernising Regulation: The New Health Professions Council*, London: Department of Health.

Department of Health (2001e) *Shifting the Balance of Power within the NHS: Securing Delivery*, London: Department of Health.

Department of Health and Social Security (1979) *Patients First*, London: HMSO.

Department of Health and Social Security (1983) *NHS Management Enquiry*, London: HMSO.

Derber, C., Schwartz, W. and Magrass, Y. (1990) *Power in the Highest Degree: Professionals and the Rise of the New Mandarin Order*, Oxford: Oxford University Press.

Dingwall, R. (1994) 'Litigation and the threat to medicine', in Gabe, J., Kelleher, D. and Williams, G. (eds) *Challenging Medicine*, London: Routledge.

Dingwall, R., Rafferty, A. and Webster, C. (1988) *An Introduction to the Social History of Nursing*, London: Routledge.

Donnison, J. (1977) *Midwives and Medical Men*, London: Heinemann.

Doyal, L. (1979) *Political Economy of Health*, London: Pluto Press.

Dubos, R. (1959) *Mirage of Health: Utopias, Progress and Biological Chance*, New York: Harper.

Duffin, J. (1999) *History of Medicine*, Toronto: University of Toronto Press.

Duffy, J. (1979) *The Healers: A History of American Medicine*, Chicago: University of Illinois Press.

Duin, N. and Sutcliffe, J. (1992) *A History of Medicine: From Prehistory to the Year 2020*, London: Simon & Schuster.

Eagle, R. (1978) *Alternative Medicine*, London: Futura.

Eckstein, H. (1960) *Pressure Group Politics: The Case of the British Medical Association*, London: Allen & Unwin.

Ehrenreich, B. and English, D. (1973) *Witches, Midwives and Nurses: A History of Women Healers*, New York: Feminist Press.

Eisenberg, D., Kessler, R., Foster, C., Norlock, F., Calkins, D. and Delbanco,

T. (1993) 'Unconventional medicine in the United States: prevalence, costs, and patterns of use', *New England Journal of Medicine*, 328: 246–52.

Eisenberg, D., Davis, R., Ettner, S., Appel, S., Wilkey, S., Rompay, M. and Kessler, R. (1998) 'Trends in alternative medicine use in the United States, 1990–1997', *Journal of the American Medical Association*, 280: 1569–75.

Elliott, P. (1972) *The Sociology of Professions*, London: Macmillan.

Ellis, H. (1997) 'Surgery and manipulation', in Porter, R. (ed.) *Medicine: A History of Healing*, London: Ivy Press.

Elston, M. A. (1991) 'The politics of professional power: medicine in a changing health service', in Gabe, J., Calnan, M. and Bury, M. (eds) *The Sociology of the Health Service*, London: Routledge.

Elston, M. A. (1994) 'The anti-vivisectionist movement and the science of medicine', in Gabe, J., Kelleher, D. and Williams, G. (eds) *Challenging Medicine*, London: Routledge.

Engel, G. (1980) 'The clinical application of the biopsychosocial model', *American Journal of Psychiatry*, 137: 535–44.

Ernst, E. (2000) 'Assessing the evidence base for CAM', in Kelner, M., Wellman, B., Pescosolido, B. and Saks, M. (eds) *Complementary and Alternative Medicine: Challenge and Change*, Amsterdam: Harwood Academic Publishers.

Ernst, E., Pittler, M., Stevinson, C. and White, A. (eds) (2001) *The Desktop Guide to Complementary and Alternative Medicine: An Evidence-based Approach*, London: Mosby.

Esquith, S. L. (1987) 'Professional authority and state power', *Theory and Society*, 16, 237–62.

Etzioni, A. (ed.) (1969) *The Semi-professions and Their Organization*, New York: Free Press.

Fereday, G. (1999) 'Community Health Councils: helping patients through the complaints procedure', in Rosenthal, M., Mulcahy, L. and Lloyd-Bostock, S. (eds) *Medical Mishaps: Pieces of the Puzzle*, Buckingham: Open University Press.

Field, M. G. (2000) 'Soviet medicine', in Cooter, R. and Pickstone, J. (eds) *Medicine in the Twentieth Century*, Amsterdam: Harwood Academic Publishers.

Fisher, P. and Ward, A. (1994) 'Complementary medicine in Europe', *British Medical Journal*, 309: 107–11.

Forsyth, G. (1966) *Doctors and State Medicine: A Study of the British Health Service*, London: Pitman Medical.

Foundation for Integrated Medicine (1997) *Integrated Healthcare*, London: FIM.

Freidson, E. (1970) *Profession of Medicine*, New York: Dodd, Mead & Co.

Freidson, E. (1986) *Professional Powers: A Study of the Institutionalization of Formal Knowledge*, Chicago: University of Chicago Press.

Freidson, E. (1989) *Medical Work in America*, New Haven, CT: Yale University Press.

Freidson, E. (1994) *Professionalism Reborn: Theory, Prophecy and Progress*, Chicago: University of Chicago Press.

Freidson, E. (2001) *Professionalism: The Third Logic*, Cambridge: Polity Press.

Friedman, M. (1962) *Capitalism and Freedom*, Chicago: University of Chicago Press.

Fry, J. (1969) *Medicine in Three Societies: A Comparison of Medical Care in the USSR, USA and UK*, Aylesbury: MTP.

Fulder, S. (1996) *The Handbook of Alternative and Complementary Medicine*, 3rd edition, Oxford: Oxford University Press.

Fulder, S. and Monro, R. (1981) *The Status of Complementary Medicine in the UK*, London: Threshold Foundation.

Furnham, A. and Vincent, C. (2000) 'Reasons for using CAM', in Kelner, M., Wellman, B., Pescosolido, B. and Saks, M. (eds) *Complementary and Alternative Medicine: Challenge and Change*, Amsterdam: Harwood Academic Publishers.

Gabe, J. and Calnan, M. (1991) 'Recent developments in general practice: a sociological analysis', in Gabe, J., Calnan, M. and Bury, M. (eds) *The Sociology of the Health Service*, London: Routledge.

Garmarnikow, E. (1978) 'Sexual divisions of labour: the case of nursing', in Kuhn, A. and Wolpe, A. M. (eds) *Feminism and Materialism*, London: Routledge & Kegan Paul.

General Medical Council (2000) *Proposals for Revalidation: Ensuring Standards, Securing the Future*, London: General Medical Council.

Gevitz, N. (1982) *The D.O.'s: Osteopathic Medicine in America*, Baltimore: Johns Hopkins University Press.

Gevitz, N. (1988a) 'Osteopathic medicine: from deviance to difference', in Gevitz, N. (ed.) *Other Healers: Unorthodox Medicine in America*, Baltimore: Johns Hopkins University Press.

Gevitz, N. (1988b) 'Three perspectives on unorthodox medicine', in Gevitz, N. (ed.) *Other Healers: Unorthodox Medicine in America*, Baltimore: Johns Hopkins University Press.

Gevitz, N. (1992) ' "But all those authors are foreigners": American literary nationalism and domestic medical guides', in Porter, R. (ed.) *The Popularization of Medicine 1650–1850*, London: Routledge.

Giddens, A. (1991) *The Consequences of Modernity*, Cambridge: Polity Press.

Gill, D. (1975) 'The British National Health Service: professional determinants of administrative structure', in Cox, C. and Mead, A. (eds) *A Sociology of Medical Practice*, London: Collier-Macmillan.

Goldstein, M. (2000) 'The culture of fitness and the growth of CAM', in Kelner, M., Wellman, B., Pescosolido, B. and Saks, M. (eds) *Complementary and Alternative Medicine: Challenge and Change*, Amsterdam: Harwood Academic Publishers.

Goode, W. (1960) 'Encroachment, charlatanism and the emerging profession: psychology, sociology and medicine', *American Sociological Review*, 25: 902–14.

Gordon, J. (1981) 'Holistic health centers', in Hastings, A., Fadiman, J. and Gordon, J. (eds) *Health for the Whole Person*, New York: Bantam Books.

Gordon, J. (1988) *Holistic Medicine*, New York: Chelsea House Publishers.

Gordon, J. (1996) *Manifesto for a New Medicine*, Reading, MA: Perseus Books.

Gould, D. (1985) *The Medical Mafia*, London: Sphere.

Griffith, B., Iliffe, S. and Rayner, G. (1987) *Banking on Sickness: Commercial Medicine in Britain and the USA*, London: Lawrence & Wishart.

Griggs, B. (1997) *New Green Pharmacy: The Story of Western Herbal Medicine*, 2nd edition, London: Vermilion.

Hacker, J. (2001) 'Learning from defeat? Political analysis and the failure of health care reform in the United States', *British Journal of Political Science*, 31: 61–94.

Hafner-Eaton, C. (1994) 'When the phoenix rises, where will she go? The women's health agenda', in Rosenau, P. V. (ed.) *Health Care Reforms in the Nineties*, Thousand Oaks, CA: Sage.

Hall, S., Held, D. and McGrew, T. (eds) (1992) *Modernity and Its Futures*, Cambridge: Polity Press.

Harrison, S., Hunter, D. and Pollitt, C. (1990) *The Dynamics of British Health Policy*, London: Unwin Hyman.

Haug, M. (1973) 'Deprofessionalization: an alternative hypothesis for the future', in Halmos, P. (ed.) *Professionalization and Social Change*, Sociological Review Monograph no. 20, Keele: University of Keele.

Haug, M. (1988) 'A re-examination of the hypothesis of physician deprofessionalization', *Milbank Quarterly*, 66: 48–56.

Heirich, M. (1998) *Rethinking Health Care: Innovation and Change in America*, Boulder, CO: Westview Press.

Hellander, I. (2001) 'A review of data on the health sector of the United States', *International Journal of Health Services*, 31: 35–53.

Helman, C. (2000) *Culture, Health and Illness*, 4th edition, London: Arnold.

Higgins, J. (1988) *The Business of Medicine: Private Health Care in Britain*, London: Macmillan.

House of Lords Select Committee on Science and Technology (2000) *Report on Complementary and Alternative Medicine*, London: The Stationery Office.

Huggon, T. and Trench, A. (1992) 'Brussels post-1992: protector or persecutor?', in Saks, M. (ed.) *Alternative Medicine in Britain*, Oxford: Clarendon Press.

Illich, I. (1976) *Limits to Medicine*, Harmondsworth: Penguin.

Inglis, B. (1980) *Natural Medicine*, London: Fontana.

Jewson, N. (1974) 'Medical knowledge and the patronage system in eighteenth century England', *Sociology*, 8: 369–85.

Jewson, N. (1976) 'The disappearance of the sick-man from medical cosmology 1770–1870', *Sociology*, 10: 225–44.

JM Consulting (1996) *The Regulation of Health Professions: Report of a Review of the Professions Supplementary to Medicine Act (1960) with Recommendations for New Legislation*, Bristol: JM Consulting.

JM Consulting (1998) *The Regulation of Nurses, Midwives and Health Visitors: Report on a Review of the Nurses, Midwives and Health Visitors Act 1997*, Bristol: JM Consulting.

Johnson, T. (1972) *Professions and Power*, London: Macmillan.

Johnson, T. (1977) 'The professions in the class structure', in Scase, R. (ed.) *Industrial Society: Class Cleavage and Control*, London: Allen & Unwin.

Johnson, T. (1980) 'Work and power', in Esland, G. and Salaman, G. (eds) *The Politics of Work and Occupations*, Milton Keynes: Open University Press.

Johnson, T. (1995) 'Governmentality and the institutionalization of expertise', in Johnson, T., Larkin, G. and Saks, M. (eds) *Health Professions and the State in Europe*, London: Routledge.

Jones, H. (1994) *Health and Society in Twentieth-Century Britain*, London: Longman.

Jones, P. (1981) *Doctors and the BMA: A Case Study in Collective Action*, Farnborough: Gower.

Kalisch, P. A. and Kalisch, B. J. (1995) *The Advance of American Nursing*, 3rd edition, Philadelphia: J. B. Lippincott.

Kaptchuk, T. and Croucher, M. (1986) *The Healing Arts: A Journey through the Faces of Medicine*, London: British Broadcasting Corporation.

Kaufman, M. (1988) 'Homeopathy in America: the rise and fall and persistence of a medical heresy', in Gevitz, N. (ed.) *Other Healers: Unorthodox Medicine in America*, Baltimore: Johns Hopkins University Press.

Kelleher, D., Gabe, J. and Williams, G. (1994) 'Understanding medical dominance in the modern world', in Gabe, J., Kelleher, D. and Williams, G. (eds) *Challenging Medicine*, London: Routledge.

Kelner, M. and Wellman, B. (1997a) 'Health care and consumer choice: medical and alternative therapies', *Social Sciences and Medicine*, 45: 203–12.

Kelner, M. and Wellman, B. (1997b) 'Who seeks alternative care? A profile of the users of five modes of treatment', *Journal of Alternative and Complementary Medicine*, 3: 127–40.

Kelner, M. and Wellman, B. (2000) 'Introduction', in Kelner, M., Wellman, B., Pescosolido, B. and Saks, M. (eds) *Complementary and Alternative Medicine: Challenge and Change*, Amsterdam: Harwood Academic Publishers.

Kingdom, J. (1996) 'The United Kingdom', in Wall, A. (ed.) *Health Care Systems in Liberal Democracies*, London: Routledge.

Kingston, J. (1976) *Healing without Medicine*, London: Aldus Books.

Klein, R. (1989) *The Politics of the National Health Service*, 2nd edition, London: Longman.

Krause, E. (1996) *Death of the Guilds: Professions, States, and the Advance of Capitalism, 1930 to the Present*, New Haven, CT: Yale University Press.

Kuhn, T. (1970) *The Structure of Scientific Revolutions*, 2nd edition, Chicago: Chicago University Press.

Laing, R. D. (1976) *The Politics of the Family*, Harmondsworth: Penguin.

Lancet (1871) 'Quackery', *Lancet*, 21 October: 598.

Lancet (1889) 'How quackery is supported', *Lancet*, 6 July: 51.

Larkin, G. (1983) *Occupational Monopoly and Modern Medicine*, London: Tavistock.

Larkin, G. (1992) 'Orthodox and osteopathic medicine in the inter-war years', in Saks, M. (ed.) *Alternative Medicine in Britain*, Oxford: Clarendon Press.

Larkin, G. (1993) 'Continuity in change: medical dominance in the United Kingdom', in Hafferty, F. and McKinlay, J. (eds) *The Changing Medical Profession: An International Perspective*, Oxford: Oxford University Press.

Larkin, G. (1995) 'State control and the health professions in the United Kingdom: historical perspectives', in Johnson, T., Larkin, G. and Saks, M. (eds) *Health Professions and the State in Europe*, London: Routledge.

Larkin, G. (2000) 'Health workers', in Cooter, R. and Pickstone, J. (eds) *Medicine in the Twentieth Century*, Amsterdam: Harwood Academic Publishers.

Larner, C. (1992) 'Healing in pre-industrial Britain', in Saks, M. (ed.) *Alternative Medicine in Britain*, Oxford: Clarendon Press.

Larson, M. (1977) *The Rise of Professionalism: A Sociological Analysis*, Berkeley: University of California Press.

Le Fanu, J. (1999) *The Rise and Fall of Modern Medicine*, London: Abacus.

Leathard, A. (ed.) (1994) *Going Inter-professional: Working Together for Health and Welfare*, London: Routledge.

Leeson, J. and Gray, J. (1978) *Women and Medicine*, London: Tavistock.

Levitt, R., Wall, A., and Appleby, J. (1995) *The Reorganized National Health Service*, 5th edition, London: Chapman & Hall.

Lewith, G. (1998) 'Misconceptions about research in complementary medicine', in Vickers, A. (ed.) *Examining Complementary Medicine*, Cheltenham: Stanley Thornes.

Lewith, G. and Aldridge, J. (1991) *Complementary Medicine and the European Community*, Saffron Walden: C. W. Daniel.

Light, D. (1993) 'Countervailing power: the changing character of the medical profession in the United States', in Hafferty, F. and McKinlay, J. (eds) *The Changing Medical Profession: An International Perspective*, Oxford: Oxford University Press.

Light, D. (1995) 'Countervailing powers: a framework for professions in transition', in Johnson, T., Larkin, G. and Saks, M. (eds) *Health Professions and the State in Europe*, London: Routledge.

Lu Gwei-Djen and Needham, J. (1980) *Celestial Lancets: A History and Rationale of Acupuncture and Moxa*, Cambridge: Cambridge University Press.

Lyng, S. (1990) *Holistic Health and Biomedical Medicine: A Countersystem Analysis*, New York: SUNY Press.

Macdonald, A. (1982) *Acupuncture: From Ancient Art to Modern Medicine*, London: Allen & Unwin.

Macdonald, K. (1985) 'Social closure and occupational registration', *Sociology*, 19: 541–56.

Macdonald, K. (1995) *The Sociology of the Professions*, London: Sage.

MacEoin, D. (1990) 'The myth of clinical trials', *Journal of Alternative and Complementary Medicine*, 8: 15–18.

McGuire, M. (1988) *Ritual Healing in Suburban America*, New Brunswick, NJ: Rutgers University Press.

McGuire, M. and Anderson, W. (1999) *The US Healthcare Dilemma: Mirrors and Chains*, Westport, CT: Auburn House.

McKee, J. (1988) 'Holistic health and the critique of Western medicine', *Social Science and Medicine*, 26: 775–84.

McKeown, T. (1979) *The Role of Medicine: Dream, Mirage or Nemesis?*, Oxford: Basil Blackwell.

McKinlay, J. (1977) 'The business of good doctoring or doctoring as good business: reflections on Freidson's view of the medical game', *International Journal of Health Services*, 7: 459–83.

McKinlay, J. (ed.) (1984) *Issues in the Political Economy of Health Care*, London: Tavistock.

McKinlay, J. and Arches, J. (1985) 'Towards the proletarianization of physicians', *International Journal of Health Services*, 15: 161–95.

McKinlay, J. and Stoeckle, J. (1988) 'Corporatization and the social transformation of doctoring', *International Journal of Health Services*, 18: 191–205.

Maioni, A. (1998) *Parting at the Crossroads: The Emergence of Health Insurance in the United States and Canada*, Princeton, NJ: Princeton University Press.

Maple, E. (1992) 'The great age of quackery', in Saks, M. (ed.) *Alternative Medicine in Britain*, Oxford: Clarendon Press.

Marcus, A. I. (1996) 'From individual practitioner to regular physician: Cincinnati medical societies and the problem of definition among mid-nineteenth century Americans', in Cravens, H., Marcus, A. I. and Katzman, D. M. (eds) *Technical Knowledge in American Culture: Science, Technology, and Medicine since the Early 1800s*, Tuscaloosa: University of Alabama Press.

Marmor, T. R. (1998) 'The procompetitive movement in American medical politics', in Ranade, W. (ed.) *Markets and Health Care: A Comparative Analysis*, Harlow: Addison Wesley Longman.

Martin, S. (1994) ' "The only true scientific method of healing": chiropractic and American science 1895–1990', *Isis*, 85: 207–27.

Meade, T. W., Dyer, S., Browne, W., Townsend, J. and Frank, A. O. (1990) 'Low back pain of mechanical origin: randomised comparison of chiropractic and hospital outpatient treatment', *British Medical Journal*, 300: 1431–7.

Merton, R. K. (1968) *Social Theory and Social Structure*, New York: Free Press.

Millerson, G. (1964) *The Qualifying Associations*, London: Routledge & Kegan Paul.

Mills, S. and Budd, S. (2000) *Professional Organisation of Complementary and Alternative Medicine in the United Kingdom: A Second Report to the Department of Health*, Exeter: University of Exeter.

Mills, S. and Peacock, W. (1997) *Professional Organisation of Complementary and Alternative Medicine in the United Kingdom: Report to the Department of Health*, Exeter: University of Exeter.

Monckton, J., Belicza, B., Betz, W., Engelbart, H. and Van Wassenhoven, M. (eds) (1998) *COST Action B4: Unconventional Medicine: Final Report of the Management Committee*, Luxembourg: Office for Official Publications of the European Communities.

Moran, M. (1999) *Governing the Health Care State: A Comparative Study of the United Kingdom, the United States and Germany*, Manchester: Manchester University Press.

Moran, M. and Wood, B. (1993) *States, Regulation and the Medical Profession*, Buckingham: Open University Press.

Morgan, D., Glanville, H., Mars, S. and Nathanson, S. (1998) 'Education and training in complementary and alternative medicine: a postal survey of UK universities, medical schools and faculties of nursing education', *Complementary Therapies in Medicine*, 6: 64–70.

Moss, N. (2000) 'Socioeconomic disparities in health in the US: an agenda for action', *Social Science and Medicine*, 51: 1627–38.

National Center for Complementary and Alternative Medicine (2001a) 'A message from the Director', *Complementary and Alternative Medicine at the NIH*, 8: 3–5.

National Center for Complementary and Alternative Medicine (2001b) 'White House Commission update', *Complementary and Alternative Medicine at the NIH*, 8: 2.

Navarro, V. (1976) *Medicine under Capitalism*, New York: Prodist.

Navarro, V. (1978) *Class Struggle, the State and Medicine: An Historical and Contemporary Analysis of the Medical Sector in Great Britain*, London: Martin Robertson.

Navarro, V. (1986) *Crisis, Health and Medicine: A Social Critique*, London: Tavistock.

Navarro, V. (ed.) (1992) *Why Does the United States Not Have a National Health Programe?*, Amityville, NY: Baywood Publishing Company.

Navarro, V. (1994) *The Politics of Health Policy: The US Reforms 1980–1994*, Oxford: Blackwell.

Nettleton, S. (1992) *Power, Pain and Dentistry*, Buckingham: Open University Press.

Nicholls, P. (1988) *Homoeopathy and the Medical Profession*, London: Croom Helm.

Oakley, A. (1992) 'The wisewoman and the doctor', in Saks, M. (ed.) *Alternative Medicine in Britain*, Oxford: Clarendon Press.

O'Connor, B. B. (2000) 'Conceptions of the body in CAM', in Kelner, M., Wellman, B., Pescosolido, B. and Saks, M. (eds) *Complementary and Alternative Medicine: Challenge and Change*, Amsterdam: Harwood Academic Publishers.

Owens, P., Carrier, J. and Horder, J. (eds) (1995) *Interprofessional Issues in Community and Primary Health Care*, London: Macmillan.

Parkin, F. (1979) *Marxism and Class Theory: A Bourgeois Critique*, London: Tavistock.

Parry, J. and Parry, N. (1976) *The Rise of the Medical Profession*, London: Croom Helm.

Parry, J. and Parry, N. (1977) 'Social closure and collective social mobility', in Scase, R. (ed.) *Industrial Society: Class Cleavage and Control*, London: Allen & Unwin.

Parsons, T. (ed.) (1954) *Essays in Sociological Theory*, London: The Free Press of Glencoe.

Parssinen, T. (1979) 'Professional deviants and the history of medicine: medical mesmerists in Victorian Britain', in Wallis, R. (ed.) *On the Margins of Science: The Social Construction of Rejected Knowledge*, Sociological Review Monograph no. 27, Keele: University of Keele.

Pavek, R. (1995) 'Current status of alternative health practices in the United States', *Contemporary Internal Medicine*, 7: 61–71.

Payer, L. (1990) *Medicine and Culture*, London: Victor Gollancz.

Peters, D. (1994) 'Sharing responsibility for patient care: doctors and complementary practitioners', in Budd, S. and Sharma, U. (eds) *The Healing Bond*, London: Routledge.

Peters, D. (1998) 'Is complementary medicine holistic?', in Vickers, A. (ed.) *Examining Complementary Medicine*, Cheltenham: Stanley Thornes.

Phillips, A. and Rakusen, J. (1989) *Our Bodies Ourselves*, Harmondsworth: Penguin.

Pietroni, P. (1991) *The Greening of Medicine*, London: Victor Gollancz.

Popper, K. (1963) *Conjectures and Refutations*, London: Routledge & Kegan Paul.

Porter, R. (1992) 'Introduction', in Porter, R. (ed.) *The Popularization of Medicine 1650–1850*, London: Routledge.

Porter, R. (1994) 'Quacks: an unconscionable time dying', in Budd, S. and Sharma, U. (eds) *The Healing Bond*, London: Routledge.

Porter, R. (1995) *Disease, Medicine and Society, 1550–1860*, 2nd edition, Cambridge: Cambridge University Press.

Porter, R. (2001) *Quacks: Fakers and Charlatans in English Medicine*, Stroud: Tempus.

Portwood, D. and Fielding, A. (1981) 'Privilege and the professions', *Sociological Review*, 29: 749–73.

Raffel, M. W. and Raffel, N. (1994) *The US Health System: Origins and Functions*, 4th edition, New York: Delmar.

Rafferty, A. M. (1996) *The Politics of Nursing Knowledge*, London: Routledge.

Rees, K. (1988) 'Water as a commodity: hydropathy in Matlock', in Cooter, R. (ed.) *Studies in the History of Alternative Medicine*, Basingstoke: Macmillan.

Report as to the Practice of Medicine and Surgery by Unqualified Persons in the United Kingdom (1910) London: HMSO.

Report of the Royal Commission on the National Health Service (1979) London: HMSO.

Rice, M. F. and Winn, M. (1991) 'Black health care and the American health system: a political perspective', in Litman, T. and Robins, L. (eds) *Health Politics and Policy*, 2nd edition, New York: Delmar.

Robinson, R. and Steiner, A. (1998) *Managed Health Care: US Evidence and Lessons for the National Health Service*, Buckingham: Open University Press.

Rodwin, M. (1996) 'Consumer protection and managed care: issues, reform proposals, and trade-offs', *Houston Law Review*, 32: 1319–81.

Roebuck, J. and Quan, R. (1976) 'Health-care practices in the American Deep South', in Wallis, R. and Morley, P. (eds) *Marginal Medicine*, London: Peter Owen.

Roemer, M. (1977) *Comparative National Policies on Health Care*, New York: Marcel Dekker.

Rosenthal, M. (1987) *Dealing with Medical Malpractice: The British and Swedish Experience*, London: Tavistock.

Roszak, T. (1970) *The Making of a Counter Culture*, London: Faber & Faber.

Rothstein, W. G. (1972) *American Physicians in the Nineteenth Century: From Sects to Science*, Baltimore: Johns Hopkins University Press.

Rothstein, W. G. (1973) 'Professionalization and employer demands: the cases of homoeopathy and psychoanalysis in the United States', in Halmos, P. (ed) *Professionalisation and Social Change*, Sociological Review Monograph no. 20, Keele: University of Keele.

Rothstein, W. G. (1988) 'The botanical movements and orthodox medicine', in Gevitz, N. (ed.) *Other Healers: Unorthodox Medicine in America*, Baltimore: Johns Hopkins University Press.

Saks, M. (1983) 'Removing the blinkers? A critique of recent contributions to the sociology of professions', *Sociological Review*, 31: 1–21.

Saks, M. (1987) 'The politics of health care', in Robins, L. (ed.) *Politics and Policy-Making in Britain*, London: Longman.

Saks, M. (1991a) 'Power, politics and alternative medicine', *Talking Politics*, 3: 68–72.

Saks, M. (1991b) 'The flight from science? The reporting of acupuncture in mainstream British medical journals from 1800 to 1990', *Complementary Medical Research*, 5: 178–82.

Saks, M. (1992a) 'Introduction', in Saks, M. (ed.) *Alternative Medicine in Britain*, Oxford: Clarendon Press.

Saks, M. (1992b) 'The paradox of incorporation: acupuncture and the medical profession in modern Britain', in Saks, M. (ed.) *Alternative Medicine in Britain*, Oxford: Clarendon Press.

Saks, M. (1994) 'The alternatives to medicine', in Gabe, J., Kelleher, D. and Williams, G. (eds) *Challenging Medicine*, London: Routledge.

Saks, M. (1995a) 'Educational and professional developments in acupuncture in Britain: an historical and contemporary overview', *European Journal of Oriental Medicine*, Winter: 32–4.

Saks, M. (1995b) *Professions and the Public Interest: Professional Power, Altruism and Alternative Medicine*, London: Routledge.

Saks, M. (1996) 'From quackery to complementary medicine: the shifting boundaries between orthodox and unorthodox medical knowledge', in Cant, S. and Sharma, U. (eds) *Complementary and Alternative Medicines: Knowledge in Practice*, London: Free Association Books.

Saks, M. (1997a) 'Alternative therapies: are they holistic?', *Complementary Therapies in Nursing and Midwifery*, 3: 4–8.

Saks, M. (1997b) 'East meets West: the emergence of a holistic tradition', in Porter, R. (ed.) *Medicine: A History of Healing*, London: Ivy Press.

Saks, M. (1998a) 'Medicine and complementary medicine: challenge and change', in Scambler, G. and Higgs, P. (eds) *Modernity, Medicine and Health*, London: Routledge.

Saks, M. (1998b) 'Professionalism and health care', in Field, D. and Taylor, S. (eds) *Sociological Perspectives on Health, Illness and Health Care*, Oxford: Blackwell Science.

Saks, M. (1999a) 'Beyond the frontiers of science? Religious aspects of alternative medicine', in Hinnells, J. R. and Porter, R. (eds) *Religion, Health and Suffering*, London: Kegan Paul International.

Saks, M. (1999b) 'The wheel turns? Professionalisation and alternative medicine in Britain', *Journal of Interprofessional Care*, 13: 129–38.

Saks, M. (1999c) 'Towards integrated health care: shifting professional interests and identities in Britain', in Hellberg, I., Saks, M. and Benoit, C. (eds) *Professional Identities in Transition: Cross-cultural Dimensions*, Södertälje, Sweden: Almqvist & Wiksell International.

Saks, M. (2000a) 'Medicine and the counter culture', in Cooter, R. and Pickstone, J. (eds) *Medicine in the Twentieth Century*, Amsterdam: Harwood Academic Publishers.

Saks, M. (2000b) 'Professionalization, politics and CAM', in Kelner, M., Wellman, B., Pescosolido, B. and Saks, M. (eds) *Complementary and Alternative Medicine: Challenge and Change*, Amsterdam: Harwood Academic Publishers.

Saks, M. (2001) 'Alternative medicine and the health care division of labour: present trends and future prospects', *Current Sociology*, 49: 119–34.

Salmon, J. W. (1985) 'Introduction', in Salmon, J. W. (ed.) *Alternative Medicines: Popular and Policy Perspectives*, London: Tavistock.

Saunders, P. (1986) *Social Theory and the Urban Question*, 2nd edition, London: Hutchinson.

Schoepflin, R. B. (1988) 'Christian Science healing in America', in Gevitz, N. (ed.) *Other Healers: Unorthodox Medicine in America*, Baltimore: Johns Hopkins University Press.

Sekhri, N. (2000) 'Managed care: the US experience', *Bulletin of the World Health Organization*, 78: 830–44.

Sharma, U. (1995) *Complementary Medicine Today: Practitioners and Patients*, revised edition, London: Routledge.

Shaw, G. B. (1975) *The Doctor's Dilemma*, Harmondsworth: Penguin.

Shearer, R. and Simpson, J. (2001) 'Introduction', in Shearer, R. and Simpson, J. (eds) *Perspectives on Complementary and Alternative Health Care*, Ottawa: Health Canada.

Shi, L. (2001) 'The convergence of vulnerable characteristics and health insurance in the US', *Social Science and Medicine*, 53: 519–29.

Stacey, M. (1985) 'Women and health: the United States and the United Kingdom compared', in Lewin, E. and Olesen, V. (eds) *Women, Health and Healing: Towards a New Perspective*, London: Tavistock.

Stacey, M. (1988) *The Sociology of Health and Healing*, London: Unwin Hyman.

Stacey, M. (1992) *Regulating British Medicine: The General Medical Council*, Chichester: Wiley.

Stalker, D. and Glymore, L. (eds) (1989) *Examining Holistic Medicine*, Buffalo, NY: Prometheus.

Standen, C. S. (1993) 'The implications of the Osteopaths Act', *Complementary Therapies in Medicine*, 1: 208–10.

Stanway, A. (1994) *Complementary Medicine: A Guide to Natural Therapies*, London: Penguin.

Starfield, B. (1997) 'The future of primary care in a managed care era', *International Journal of Health Services*, 27: 687–96.

Starfield, B. and Oliver, T. (1999) 'Primary care in the United States and its precarious future', *Health and Social Care in the Community*, 7: 315–23.

Starr, P. (1982) *The Social Transformation of American Medicine*, New York: Basic Books.

Stevens, R. (1966) *Medical Practice in Modern England*, New Haven, CT: Yale University Press.

Stevens, R. (1971) *American Medicine and the Public Interest*, New Haven, CT: Yale University Press.

Stevens, R. (1983) 'Comparisons in health care: Britain as a contrast to the United States', in Mechanic, D. (ed.) *Handbook of Health, Health Care and Health Professions*, New York: Free Press.

Stevens, R. (1986) 'The future of the medical profession', in Ginsberg, E. (ed.) *From Physician Shortage to Patient Shortage: The Uncertain Future of Medical Practice*, Boulder, CO: Westview.

Stone, J. and Mathews, J. (1996) *Complementary Medicine and the Law*. Oxford: Oxford University Press.

Strong, P. and Robinson, J. (1990) *The NHS: Under New Management*, Milton Keynes: Open University Press.

Sullivan, K. (2001) 'On the "efficiency" of managed care plans', *International Journal of Health Services*, 31: 55–65.

Szasz, T. (1970) *The Manufacture of Madness*, New York: Harper & Row.

Taylor, C. (1995) *Myths of the North American Indians*, London: Laurence King.

Taylor, R. (1985) 'Alternative medicine and the medical encounter in Britain and the United States', in Salmon, J. W. (ed.) *Alternative Medicines: Popular and Policy Perspectives*, London: Tavistock.

Thomas, K., Carr, J., Westlake, L. and Williams, B. (1991) 'Use of non-orthodox and conventional health care in Great Britain', *British Medical Journal*, 302: 207–10.

Thomas, K., Fall, M., Parry, G. and Nicholl, J. (1995) *National Survey of Access to Complementary Health Care via General Practice: Report to the Department of Health*, Sheffield: University of Sheffield.

Thomson, A. (1973) *Half a Century of Medical Research: Origins and Policy of the Medical Research Council (UK)*, vol. 1, London: HMSO.

Toren, N. (1975) 'Deprofessionalization and its sources', *Sociology of Work and Occupations*, 2: 323–37.

Tovey, P. (1997) 'Contingent legitimacy: UK alternative practitioners and inter-sectoral acceptance', *Social Science and Medicine*, 45: 1129–33.

Townsend, P. and Davidson, N. (1982) *Inequalities in Health: The Black Report*, Harmondsworth: Penguin.

Trevelyan, J. and Booth, B. (1994) *Complementary Medicine for Nurses, Midwives and Health Visitors*, London: Macmillan.

Turner, B. (1995) *Medical Power and Social Knowledge*, 2nd edition, London: Sage.

United States Department of Health and Human Services (1985) *Report of the Secretary's Task Force on Black and Minority Health*, Washington, DC: USGPO.

United States Department of Health and Human Services (2000) *Healthy People 2010*, Washington, DC: USGPO.

Valente, T. (2000) 'Social networks and mass media: the "diffusion" of CAM', in Kelner, M., Wellman, B., Pescosolido, B. and Saks, M. (eds) *Complementary and Alternative Medicine: Challenge and Change*, Amsterdam: Harwood Academic Publishers.

Vaughan, P. (1959) *Doctors' Commons: A Short History of the British Medical Association*, London: Heinemann.

Versluis, A. (1993) *The Elements of Native American Traditions*, Shaftesbury: Element Books.

Vincent, J. (1992) 'Self-help groups and health care in contemporary Britain', in Saks, M. (ed.) *Alternative Medicine in Britain*, Oxford: Clarendon Press.

Waddington, I. (1984) *The Medical Profession in the Industrial Revolution*, London: Gill & Macmillan.

Walby, S. and Greenwell, J. (1994) *Medicine and Nursing: Professions in a Changing Health Service*, London: Sage.

Walker, M. (1994) *Dirty Medicine: Science, Big Business and the Assault on Natural Health Care*, London: Slingshot Publications.

Wallis, R. and Morley, P. (1976) 'Introduction', in Wallis, R. and Morley, P. (eds) *Marginal Medicine*, London: Peter Owen.

Wardwell, W. (1976) 'Orthodox and unorthodox practitioners: changing relationships and the future status of chiropractors', in Wallis, R. and Morley, P. (eds) *Marginal Medicine*, London: Peter Owen.

Wardwell, W. (1988) 'Chiropractors: evolution to acceptance', in Gevitz, N. (ed.) *Other Healers: Unorthodox Medicine in America*, Baltimore: Johns Hopkins University Press.

Wardwell, W. (1992) *Chiropractic: History and Evolution of a New Profession*, St Louis: Mosby.

Wardwell, W. (1994a) 'Alternative medicine in the United States', *Social Science and Medicine*, 38: 1061–8.

Wardwell, W. (1994b) 'Differential evolution of the osteopathic and chiropractic professions in the United States', *Perspectives in Biology and Medicine*, 37: 595–607.

Warner, J. H. (1987) 'Medical sectarianism, therapeutic conflict, and the shaping of orthodox professional identity in antebellum American medicine', in Bynum, W. F. and Porter, R. (eds) *Medical Fringe and Medical Orthodoxy 1750–1850*, London: Croom Helm.

Weiss, L. D. (1997) *Private Medicine and Public Health: Profit, Politics and Prejudice in the American Health Care Enterprise*, Boulder, CO: Westview Press.

White House Commission on Complementary and Alternative Medicine Policy (2002), Washington, DC: The Commission.

Whitehead, M. (1987) *The Health Divide*, London: Health Education Council.

Whorton, J. C. (1988) 'Patient, heal thyself: popular health reform movements as unorthodox medicine', in Gevitz, N. (ed.) *Other Healers: Unorthodox Medicine in America*, Baltimore: Johns Hopkins University Press.

Wilensky, H. (1964) 'The professionalization of everyone?', *American Journal of Sociology*, 70: 137–58.

Williams, S. and Calnan, M. (1996) 'Modern medicine and the lay populace: theoretical perspectives and the lay populace', in Williams, S. and Calnan, M. (eds) *Modern Medicine: Lay Perspectives and Experiences*, London: UCL Press.

Williams, S. and Popay, J. (1994) 'Lay knowledge and the privilege of experience', in Gabe, J., Kelleher, D. and Williams, G. (eds) *Challenging Medicine*, London: Routledge.

Wilson, P. (1997) 'Healers in history', in Porter, R. (ed.) *Medicine: A History of Healing*, London: Ivy Press.

Witz, A. (1992) *Professions and Patriarchy*, London: Routledge.

Witz, A. (1994) 'The challenge of nursing', in Gabe, J., Kelleher, D. and Williams, G. (eds) *Challenging Medicine*, London: Routledge.

Wolpe, P. R. (1994) 'The dynamics of heresy in a profession', *Social Science and Medicine*, 39: 1133–48.

Wright, P. (1992) 'Astrology in seventeenth-century England', in Saks, M. (ed.) *Alternative Medicine in Britain*, Oxford: Clarendon Press.

Youngson, A. (1979) *The Scientific Revolution in Victorian Medicine*, London: Croom Helm.

Index

American Medical Association 32, 33,
    34–5, 40, 55, 56, 57, 58, 59, 80, 81,
    82, 85, 86, 87, 88, 92, 101, 102, 103,
    105, 106, 120, 121, 122, 135, 136,
    137, 138, 148, 151
American Nursing Association 138
American Osteopathic Association 78
American Pharmaceutical
    Association 32
American Society of Allied Health
    Professions 102–3
American Society of Medical
    Technologists 103
amputations 12
anaesthesiology 12, 59, 61, 138
anatomy 22, 118
antibiotics 50
anti-depressants 94
antisepsis 12, 57
apothecaries 11, 12, 13–14, 15, 16, 19,
    25, 26, 37
    see also Apothecaries Act; Society of
        Apothecaries; surgeon-apothecaries;
        Worshipful Society of Apothecaries
Apothecaries Act (1815) 26
aromatherapy 2, 111, 149, 157
asepsis 42
astrology 8, 12, 14
Auenbrugger, Les 13
Avicenna 8
Ayurvedic Medicine 157, 161

barber-surgeons 19
Barker, Herbert 76
Baunscheidtism 70
Beddoes' Pneumatic Institute 14
Belgium 160
Bernard, Claude 50
Beveridge Report 49
biofeedback 2
bleeding 20, 32, 42
blistering 14
bloodletting 8, 9, 11, 14, 20
Blue Cross 57, 99, 137
Blue Shield 99

bonesetting 12, 21, 76
Britain
    deprofessionalization of medicine
        127, 139–44
    development of alternative
        medicine 66–77, 103–4, 111–19,
        148–50, 157–8, 160, 161–2
    evolution of health care system 8–17,
        48–55, 95–8, 125–31
    political system 1
    professionalization of allied health
        professions 52–5, 60, 61, 97–8,
        128, 129–30, 131
    professionalization of medicine
        24–8, 37–8, 41–2, 43–4, 45–6, 47,
        48–52, 66–7, 90, 91, 92, 128–9, 139
    self-help 108–11, 116, 151
    see also British health organizations
British Acupuncture Accreditation
    Board 149
British Acupuncture Association and
    Register 149
British Acupuncture Council 149
British Chiropractic Association 150
British Complementary Medicine
    Association 149
British Health and Freedom Society 76
British and Incorporated Associations of
    Osteopaths 75
British Medical Association 26, 52, 68,
    72, 73, 97, 103, 104, 116, 117, 118,
    141, 144
    see also Provincial Medical and
        Surgical Association
British Postgraduate Medical Federation
    77
Buchan, William 24

Campaign Against Health Fraud 118
Canada 111, 160, 162
    see also Health Canada
Cancer Act (1939) 73
cancer screening 127
cardiology 96
care technologists 138